From

JUNK FOOD

to

JOY FOOD

ALL THE FOODS
YOU LOVE TO EAT . . .
ONLY BETTER

JOY BAUER, M.S., R.D.N., C.D.N.

HAY HOUSE, INC.
Carlsbad, California ▪ New York City
London ▪ Sydney ▪ Johannesburg
Vancouver ▪ Hong Kong ▪ New Delhi

Published and distributed in the United States by: Hay House, Inc.:
www.hayhouse.com® • ***Published and distributed in Australia by:***
Hay House Australia Pty. Ltd.: www.hayhouse.com.au • ***Published
and distributed in the United Kingdom by:*** Hay House UK, Ltd.:
www.hayhouse.co.uk • ***Published and distributed in the Republic
of South Africa by:*** Hay House SA (Pty), Ltd.: info@hayhouse.co.za •
Distributed in Canada by: Raincoast Books: www.raincoast.com •
Published in India by: Hay House Publishers India: www.hayhouse.co.in

INDEXER: Laura Ogar

COVER AND INTERIOR DESIGN: Celia Fuller-Vels

Library of Congress Cataloging-in-Publication Data

Names: Bauer, Joy, author.
Title: From junk food to joy food : all the foods you love to eat . . . only
 better / Joy Bauer.
Description: 1st edition. | Carlsbad, California : Hay House, Inc., [2016] |
 Includes index.
Identifiers: LCCN 2015039438 | ISBN 9781401950378 (hardcover :
alk. paper)
Subjects: LCSH: Cooking. | Comfort food. | Quick and easy cooking. | Junk
 food. | LCGFT: Cookbooks.
Classification: LCC TX714 .B37865 2016 | DDC 641.5--dc23 LC record
available at http://lccn.loc.gov/2015039438

Hardcover ISBN: 978-1-4019-5037-8

10 9 8 7 6 5 4 3

1st edition, February 2016

PRINTED IN THE UNITED STATES OF AMERICA

SUSTAINABLE FORESTRY INITIATIVE
Certified Chain of Custody
Promoting Sustainable Forestry
www.sfiprogram.org
SFI-01268
SFI label applies to the text stock

Unless noted below, photography was done by.

PHOTOGRAPHER: Lucy Schaeffer
FOOD STYLIST: Allison Simpson
PROP STYLIST: Molly Fitzsimons

Additional photography is used under license from:

Dreamstime.com: page 28
iStock.com: pages 12, 25, 110, and 131
Joy Bauer: pages viii, 2, 62, 68, 80, 176, 194, 196, 204, and 222
Shutterstock.com: Pages 6–8, 14, 16, 18, 20, 22, 24, 26, 30, 32, 36,
38, 40–42, 44, 46, 48, 50–52, 54, 58, 64, 66, 70, 72, 74, 76, 78, 82,
84, 86, 90, 92, 94–96, 98, 100–102, 104, 106, 108, 112, 113, 115,
116, 118, 122, 126, 128, 130, 132, 134, 136, 138, 140, 142, 143,
146, 154, 156, 158, 159, 160, 162, 164, 166, 168, 172, 174, 178,
180, 182–184, 186, 188, 190–192, 198–202, 208–210, 213, 214,
216, 218, 224, 225, 228, 230–236, 238–244, 246, 248, 250, and 251
Thinkstock.com: pages 10, 60, 114, 120, 144, 149, 151, 206, 212,
220, and 237

To Ian, my amazing husband, who is my biggest supporter and best friend.
To my three beautiful children, Jesse, Cole, and Ayden Jane, who surprise me every single day.
To my favorite furry Bauer, Gatsby, who follows me around like I'm Beyoncé.

You are my everything . . . my heart, my bliss, my home, my loves.

CONTENTS

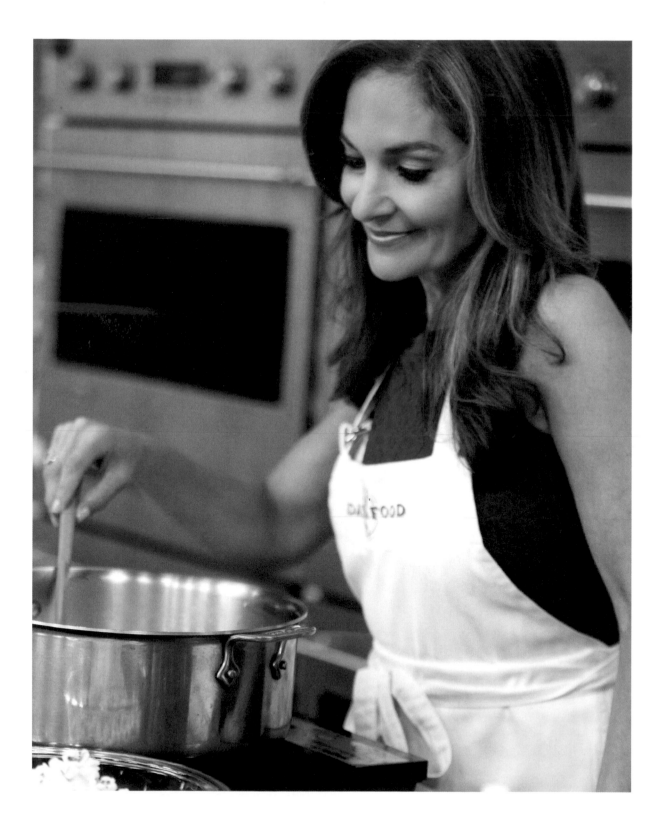

WELCOME TO MY KITCHEN

Imagine eating all the foods you love—General Tso's chicken, buffalo wings, cheese pizza, bacon cheeseburgers, strawberry cheesecake, and chocolate chip ice cream—but instead of making you feel bloated, heavy, lethargic, and guilty, what if they made you feel lighter, energized, and healthy?

Talk about a dieter's dream come true: The recipes in this book accomplish just that. On the following pages, I share the secrets to transforming your favorite junk foods into Joy Foods. With just a few simple tweaks, you'll be able to eat your favorite comfort foods—the ones that make you weak in the knees and cause your mouth to water—while losing weight, alleviating arthritis pain, boosting energy, enhancing heart health, normalizing blood pressure, flattening out your midsection, minimizing wrinkles . . . the list of benefits goes on and on. This book is packed with recipes for the most delicious (and typically fattening!) meals, snacks, desserts, and drinks—but with a healthy twist.

Why would you give up the stuff you love when you don't have to? There's no fun in following a program that forbids all the tasty comfort foods you crave. The truth is, that's the reason most diets fail. We all know what we *should* be eating, but we simply can't bypass barbecue ribs and baked beans. We can't forego fettuccine Alfredo and French onion soup. That's why issues like obesity, hypertension, high cholesterol, type 2 diabetes, and arthritis are so common. The fact is that these foods, as we know and love them, send our health into a tailspin.

Fortunately, I've found ways to lighten the bites you can't live without—the ones that you remember fondly from your childhood, the ones you could never part with as an adult—so you can enjoy them without undoing your diet. These slimmer spins on classic recipes will have your taste buds humming and party guests clamoring for a repeat invite.

That's what this entire book is about, and it was the whole idea behind my "From Junk Food to Joy Food" series, which launched on the *Today* show this past year. No more existing on plain boiled chicken, steamed broccoli, and rabbit-food salads in an effort to lose weight and get your health under control. You can continue to eat what you love by simply preparing these foods in a better-for-you way. It's like I've waved a magic health wand over all the unhealthy stuff you can't live without.

But it gets even better. Most of these recipes are a snap to prepare and include everyday ingredients you probably already have in your fridge and pantry. Most people are completely overscheduled, and the last thing I want to do is burden you with meals that take hours to make. I'm a mom of three kids with a full-time job trying to juggle work responsibilities, carpooling, and a crazy-busy home life, so I get it. I'm in the same boat, so I've gone out of my way to make things as simple as possible.

As you flip through the recipes, you can feel confident knowing that these dishes have been tested on kids, teens, and adults, and are guaranteed to be a huge hit. Everyone will be asking for seconds, and because these recipes are so much lighter than the originals, you can feel good about dishing them out.

Not only will your taste buds be happy once you sample these decadent remakes, but you will also feel markedly better. You will notice a drop on the scale and an increase in your energy levels. No deprivation or dieting required. No falling off the wagon. No guilt or regret. Your only job is to indulge and enjoy. Yes, you can now have your cake and eat it, too. So get ready to dig into all the mouthwatering recipes you love . . . only better.

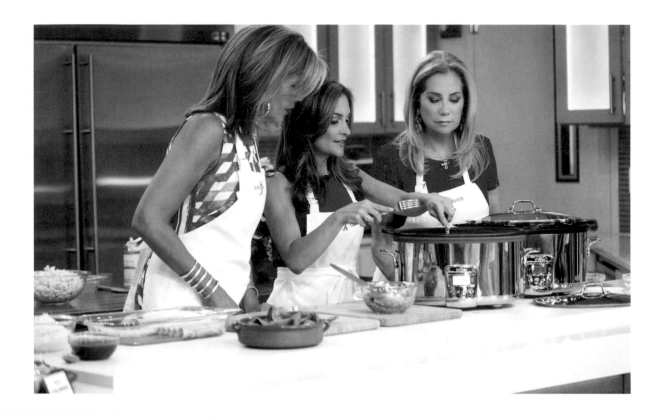

HOW TO USE THIS BOOK

I've separated this book into eight categories, which include breakfasts; dips and apps; soups and sandwiches; sides, salads, and dressings; simple suppers; pizzas and pastas; desserts; and drinks. (No surprise the dessert section is the longest—in fact, it's double the length of some of the others—as I have a *huge* sweet tooth.) You can search for a specific recipe by category or just flip through until you find something you like . . . I'm guessing that won't take too long.

You may be wondering where the *before* calories listed for each recipe come from. In some instances, it was a no-brainer—I used the figures from the most popular brand. In other cases, my team used an average of data from popular restaurant chains and/or national brand-name products, or even classic homemade recipes. As you probably know, calories vary from version to version, so I went with a fair

average after a comprehensive evaluation. In any event, the *before* numbers will provide a startling reality check about what you've been pumping into your body. The impressive *after* numbers (often including significantly fewer calories and less sugar, sodium, and saturated fat) will get you pumped to make my dishes over and over again.

In terms of portions, the *before* and *after* are usually fair swaps—one stack of pancakes for the same size stack, for example. However, we all know that restaurants are notorious for their ginormous portions, so in some cases, I made the Joy Food serving sizes more appropriate. Don't worry . . . my healthier servings are just as satisfying. If you have a hearty appetite and want more food, you can enjoy a second helping and still end up taking in far fewer calories than the traditional version.

MY FAVORITE KITCHEN GADGETS

Ready to get cooking? Before you do, I recommend investing in a few key gadgets, which will help you save time and make meal prep a snap. You'll find most of these mentioned throughout the book. Of course, having a good set of pots, pans, knives, and cutting boards is a must. Happy cooking!

- **Refillable oil mister:** This allows you to sauté veggies, lean protein, and other ingredients without adding many fat calories to recipes. Use the gadget to coat a skillet evenly with oil or to mist your veggies or a salad. I have a few misters, and I fill each one with a different healthy oil, as well as balsamic or other flavored vinegars. You can use this whenever a recipe calls for nonstick oil spray. For these recipes, I would suggest using olive oil, canola oil, or grapeseed oil.

- **Measuring cups and spoons:** These are essential for measuring spices, fats, flours, and other ingredients. I have quite the collection in my kitchen, but keeping them organized and accessible is key. In my house, they seem to disappear like socks.

- **Blender and/or food processor:** You can literally chop minutes off food prep with either of these tools. It makes chopping, shredding, and mincing large quantities a cinch. For most people, a 4- to 7-cup processor does the trick, and it won't take up too much precious counter or cabinet space.

- **Immersion (or handheld) blender:** This is great for making pureed soups or sauces because you can skip the step of transferring hot liquids to a blender in batches. (Love gadgets that save you time!)

- **Slow cooker:** This is a must-have for busy parents. Simply toss all the ingredients into the slow cooker in the morning, and when dinnertime rolls around, a delicious, wholesome meal is waiting for you. You can use it for soups, stews, and chilies.

- **Onion goggles:** Slicing an onion can be a real tearjerker. That's because the onion releases a sulfur compound that may irritate your eyes and cause them to water. I recently invested in a pair of onion goggles (about $20 at most home-goods stores) to protect my eyes . . . and fingers (let's face it, misty eyes and a sharp knife are not a good combo). You may want to do the same if you often cook with onions. (Budget-saving trick: if you have a pair of ski goggles lying around, these work just as well.)

- **Cupcake tins (various sizes):** If you bake often, these are a great investment. I love mini-cupcake tins, which are terrific for bite-size treats—automatic portion control so you don't have to rely on willpower. You can go the other direction and grab a jumbo tin, which you can use for large muffins and tasty frittatas. And don't limit standard muffin tins to just baked goods. I use mine to create mini meatloaves . . . with sweet-potato frosting.

- **Spiral slicer:** In several of my recipes, I use zucchini noodles (or "zoodles") to take the place of standard starchy pasta. To get perfect zoodles, I recommend a spiral slicer. There are various types at various price points—choose one that suits your budget. And in a pinch, you can also always use a vegetable peeler to make julienned vegetable noodles.

Wishing you good health and delicious food,

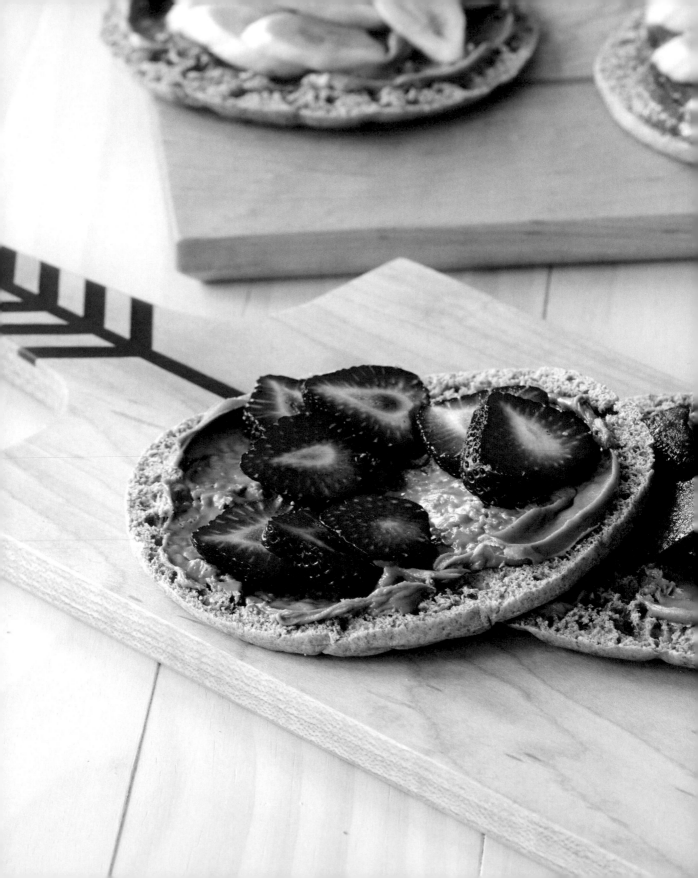

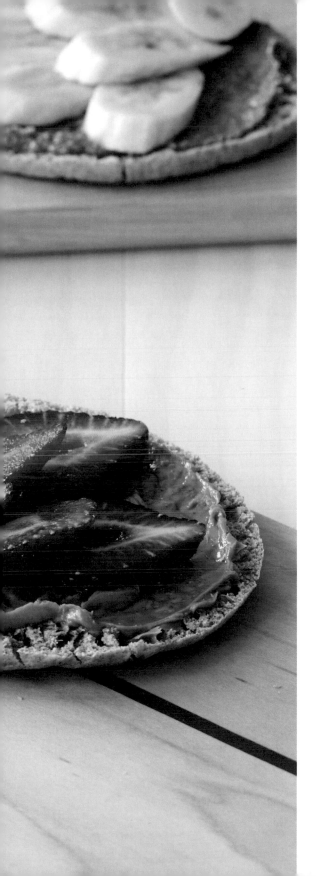

Chapter 1

BETTER-FOR-YOU BREAKFASTS

What you sprinkle in your bowl or put on your plate in the morning can have a huge impact on the rest of your day. Begin with a healthful breakfast, and you'll soar through the A.M. hours feeling focused and sharp, hunger in check, energy levels high, and productivity at its peak. Forget about good morning—we're talking *great* morning!

The breakfast recipes on the following pages include slimmer spins on the classic items we love to gobble down (think pancakes, oatmeal, French toast, ham and cheese omelets, toaster pastries, and more). These remakes will help you power through your day, and they taste absolutely delicious—I'm talking lick your fingers, dog-ear these pages, Facebook your friends delicious. So jump in and get started on the right foot with some of your favorite but *totally* health-ified breakfast foods.

Junk Food

1,000 CALORIES

EGGS BENEDICT

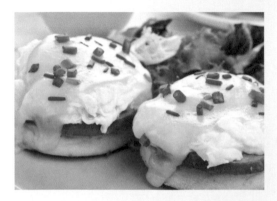

Believe it or not, many of the ingredients in this classic breakfast dish, including the egg and Canadian bacon, are actually fairly lean. The trouble is in the topping: the creamy hollandaise sauce, which is made from egg yolks and plenty of butter.

My skinny version features a secret ingredient that gives the sauce a delicious flavor and preserves its signature yellow hue: yellow bell pepper. I serve the sandwich on a whole-grain English muffin to get a bit more fiber, but if you want to dramatically cut carbs and calories, you can skip the bread and serve it on a grilled portobello mushroom cap instead.

Joy Food

377 CALORIES

EGGS BENEDICT

makes 2 servings

I created a slimmer substitute for caloric hollandaise sauce by using a creamy combination of yellow bell pepper and light or reduced-fat cream cheese. It's a delicious dish for a lazy Sunday brunch or whenever you're craving this breakfast favorite . . . like tomorrow morning.

HOLLANDAISE SAUCE
1 yellow bell pepper, seeded and cut into eighths
3 ounces (6 tablespoons) light or reduced-fat cream cheese
1 teaspoon lemon juice
½ teaspoon Dijon mustard
¼ teaspoon kosher salt or coarse sea salt

EGGS BENEDICT
4 slices Canadian bacon
1 ripe tomato, cut into 4 thick slices
1 teaspoon distilled white vinegar
4 eggs, at room temperature
2 whole-grain English muffins, halved
Paprika

To make the hollandaise: Place the bell pepper in a microwave-safe bowl and add 1 tablespoon water. Cover and microwave on high for 2 minutes or until the pepper is easily pierced with a paring knife. Drain and immediately transfer it to a blender.

Add the cream cheese, lemon juice, mustard, and salt to the blender. Puree until the sauce is silky smooth with no visible bits of yellow pepper. Set aside.

To make the Eggs Benedict: Preheat the broiler. Line a baking sheet with aluminum foil and coat with nonstick oil spray.

Arrange the Canadian bacon and tomato slices in a single layer on the prepared baking sheet. Broil for 4 minutes. Flip the bacon and tomato slices over and

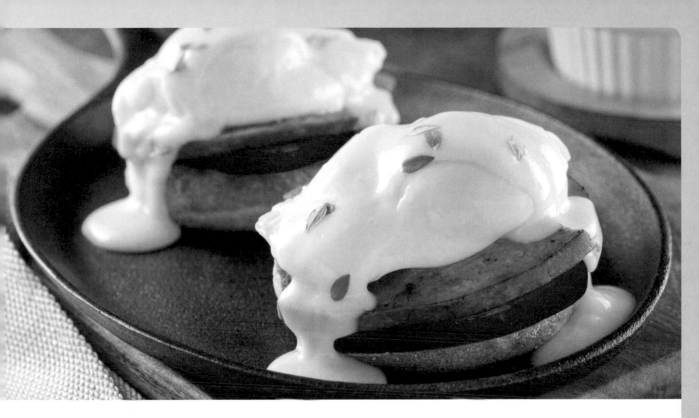

broil for 4 more minutes, or until the bacon is crispy brown around the edges. Remove the baking sheet from oven and loosely tent it with foil to keep it warm.

Place a double layer of paper towels on a platter or small baking sheet; this will be used to hold the poached eggs once they are cooked.

Fill a large shallow pan with 3 inches of water. Bring the water to a boil. Reduce the heat to low so the water is at a gentle simmer. Add the vinegar and stir.

Crack each egg into its own small bowl or container. (For best results, use containers with narrow bases and wide tops to help the eggs keep their shape. Teacups work well.) Place all the containers close to the stove.

Slip each egg carefully into the simmering water by lowering the lip of each small container or cup half an inch below the surface of the water.

When all four eggs are in the water, use a slotted spoon to gently nudge the egg whites closer to the egg yolks by swirling the water around them in a circle as they cook. For medium-firm yolks, cook for 3 minutes. (Adjust the time for runnier or firmer yolks,

cooking no more than 5 minutes.) To tell if the yolk is cooked to your liking, remove an egg from the water with a slotted spoon and gently press on the yolk to determine the degree of doneness. Remove the cooked eggs from the water with a slotted spoon and transfer them to the paper-towel-lined platter.

Just before assembling the Eggs Benedict sandwiches, toast the English muffin halves and reheat the hollandaise in a small saucepan, stirring over low heat for a few minutes, or in the microwave for 30 to 60 seconds, until it's warm to the touch.

To assemble, place a slice of tomato on each toasted English muffin half, and top with 1 slice Canadian bacon, 1 poached egg, and 1 tablespoon hollandaise sauce. Sprinkle paprika over the sauce for a pretty pop of color. Each serving includes 2 English muffin halves layered with Canadian bacon, tomato, egg, and sauce.

nutrition information PER SERVING
377 calories ▪ 29 g protein ▪ 15 g total fat (10 g unsaturated, 5 g saturated) ▪ 400 mg cholesterol ▪ 31 g carbs ▪ 4.5 g fiber 5 g total sugar (5 g natural, 0 g added) ▪ 850 mg sodium

Junk Food

750 CALORIES

DINER PANCAKES

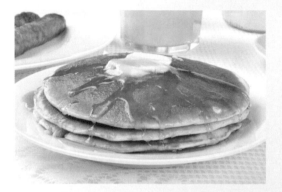

Have you seen the size of most diner-style flapjacks? They're usually creeping close to the edge of the plate. Not to mention, they're made with junky white flour—three large ones can be like eating six slices of white bread. And the toppings only make matters worse: butter packs on fat, and a typical quarter-cup pour of gooey syrup adds 12 teaspoons of straight sugar—and an extra 240 calories—to your breakfast. That makes 750 calories per order.

My Protein Pancakes are super-popular in the Bauer house, and my kids are constantly trying all sorts of tasty variations (adding blueberries, chopped nuts, even occasional semisweet chocolate chips). And because this recipe calls for just five simple ingredients, you can whip it together in just a few minutes. Plus, it's packed with energizing protein to get you going. Good morning, indeed!

> **CHOOSE IT TO LOSE IT** Make this pancake swap twice a week and you'll save more than 49,000 calories annually, which could help you shed more than 14 pounds by the end of the year.

Joy Food

270 CALORIES

PROTEIN PANCAKES

makes 1 serving

Forget carb-heavy, waist-busting flapjacks! These pancakes are full of high-quality protein from the egg whites, a smart choice if you're looking to lose weight or rev your system. They're also gluten-free and a cinch to put together.

½ cup quick-cooking oats
4 egg whites
½ teaspoon vanilla extract
1 tablespoon sugar or sugar substitute
½ teaspoon cinnamon (optional)

Generously coat a skillet with nonstick oil spray and warm over medium heat.

Combine all the ingredients in a small bowl and stir until thoroughly mixed.

Pour the mixture onto the skillet to make either 1 jumbo pancake or 5 small pancakes. Cook until you see small bubbles forming, 2 to 3 minutes for the jumbo pancake or 1 to 2 for the small pancakes. Then flip the pancake(s) over and cook until golden brown, 1 to 2 minutes.

---

nutrition information PER SERVING
270 calories ▪ 19.5 g protein ▪ 3 g total fat (2.5 g unsaturated, 0.5 g saturated) ▪ 0 mg cholesterol ▪ 41 g carbs ▪ 4 g fiber 13 g total sugar (1 g natural, 12 g added) ▪ 220 mg sodium

> **TASTY TWIST** Amp up the nutrition and flavor by mixing fruit right into the batter. Half a cup of chopped fruit is only 40 extra calories and provides an additional 2 grams of fiber. Also, try my simple trick: Nuke frozen fruit in the microwave, then pour the fruit and all the natural juices over the finished pancake as I've done in this picture. Tastes amazing . . . and no added sugar. Two more 40-calorie add-ons: ⅓ cup nonfat or low-fat yogurt or 1 teaspoon drizzle of maple syrup.

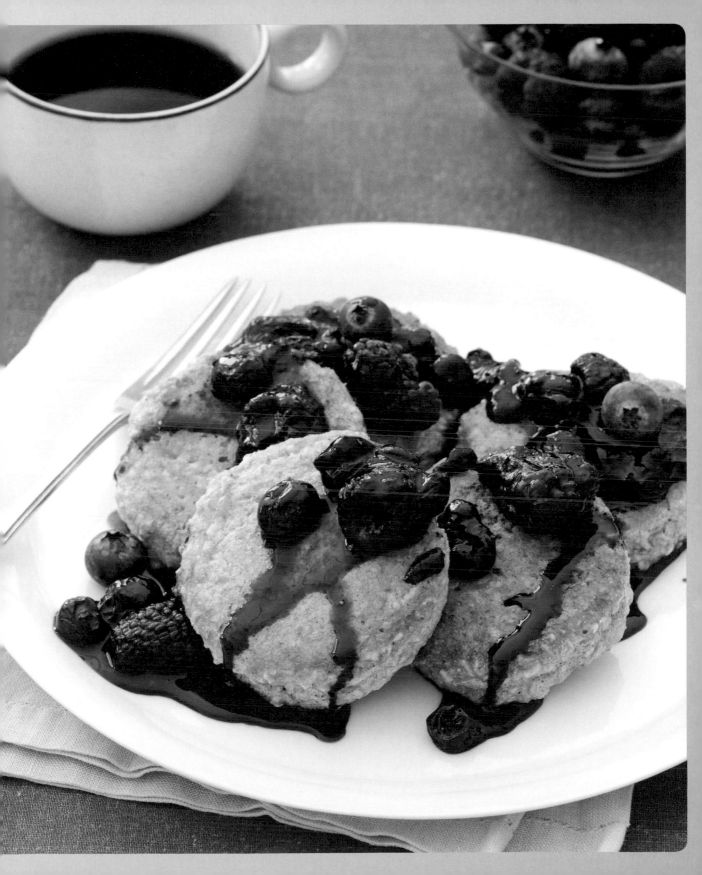

Junk Food

650 CALORIES

SILVER DOLLAR PANCAKES

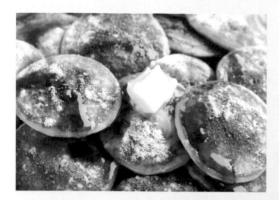

Good things come in small packages—unless they're refined, starchy, and drowning in butter and syrup. Check this out: A standard "naked" stack of silver dollar pancakes will run you about 310 calories. Top them off with the typical quarter cup of syrup and tablespoon of butter and we're talking 650 calories—you'll have to walk more than six miles to burn those "petite" babies off!

Luckily, I found an easy way to lighten up my minis so they're yummy *and* guilt-free. The best part: you won't feel weighed down when you're done eating.

Joy Food

162 CALORIES

SILVER DOLLAR PANCAKES

makes 5 servings

Presenting my marvelous minis. There's no need to finish off these flapjacks with sugary syrup or other toppings—they're sweet enough as is thanks to the creamy bananas and toasty, buttery pecans. They're also gluten-free, plus they get a shot of protein from the cottage cheese (which your finicky eaters will not taste, shhh). Dig in and enjoy!

1 cup quick-cooking oats
½ cup fat-free cottage cheese
1 ripe banana
2 eggs
1 teaspoon baking powder
1 teaspoon vanilla extract
1 teaspoon cinnamon
3 tablespoons unsweetened vanilla almond milk
¼ cup pecan halves, toasted and
    roughly chopped

Combine all ingredients, except pecans, in a blender and process until smooth.

Spray a griddle with nonstick oil spray and warm over medium-high heat.

Carefully ladle batter onto the griddle to form about 20 three-inch pancakes (about 2 tablespoons batter per pancake). Sprinkle a few pecan pieces onto each and cook until bubbles form throughout the pancakes, about 30 seconds. Flip and cook until golden brown.

---

nutrition information PER SERVING OF 4 PANCAKES
162 calories ▪ 8.5 g protein ▪ 7 g total fat (6 g unsaturated, 1 g saturated) ▪ 75 mg cholesterol ▪ 18 g carbs ▪ 3 g fiber 4 g total sugar (4 g natural, 0 g added) ▪ 210 mg sodium

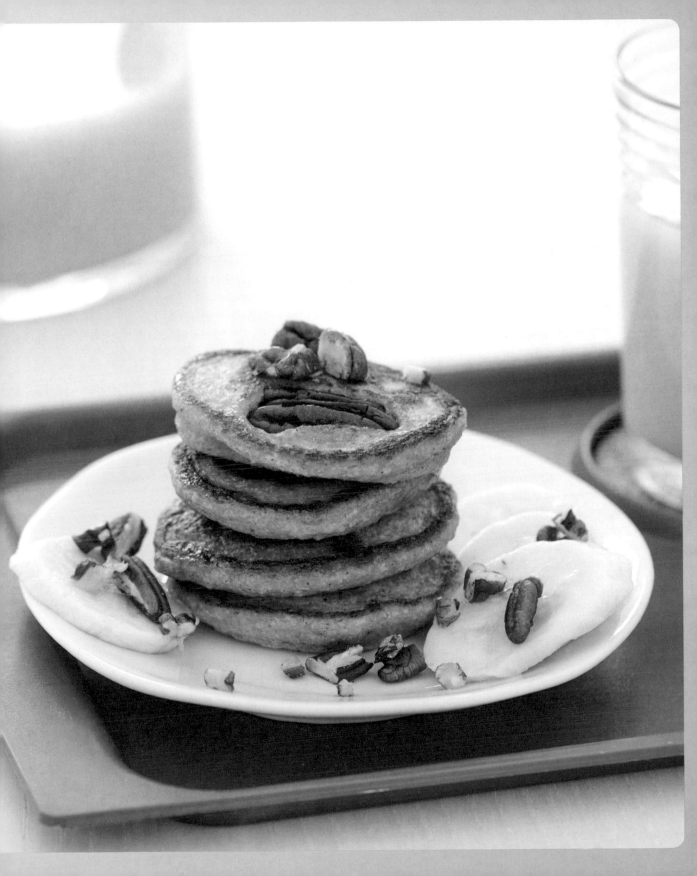

Junk Food

968 CALORIES

CHOCOLATE CHIP PANCAKES

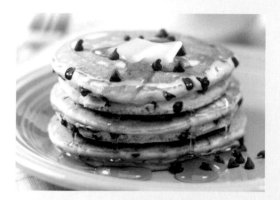

I'm a firm believer that almost everything is better with chocolate—but an order of chocolate chip pancakes from a diner might be the one exception. These overly sweetened fat bombs disguised as breakfast can actually cost you more than most desserts. At one popular pancake house, chocolate chip pancakes topped with butter and syrup clock in at 968 calories and about 78 grams of sugar. Ouch! That's more calories and sugar than two scoops of chocolate ice cream covered in hot fudge and whipped cream.

My recipe involves a few sneaky ingredients (of course) to pump up the nutrition value without compromising the taste—and you'll see, there's still plenty of chocolate to satisfy even the sweetest sweet tooth. I serve mine with canned whipped topping and dark chocolate shavings. They're fun and festive, and you'll fall in love at first bite.

Joy Food

275 CALORIES

DOUBLE CHOCOLATE CHIP PANCAKES

makes 6 servings

I knew I had struck gold when my youngest daughter, Ayden Jane, requested these pancakes for her birthday breakfast. Birthdays are very big deals in my house—I'll whip up anything the kids crave (seriously, anything). Thus, when one of their birthday requests is a Joy Food, I'm giddy with delight. Fortunately these chocolatey gems have such wholesome ingredients, you don't have to wait for a special day to prepare them. You can have these pancakes sizzling on the griddle the morning after a sleepover, before a big exam, or on a rainy Wednesday when you just feel like having chocolate for breakfast.

½ cup whole-grain flour
½ cup all-purpose flour
¼ cup unsweetened cocoa powder
¼ cup sugar
2 tablespoons ground flaxseed
1½ teaspoons baking powder
½ teaspoon salt
1 egg
1 egg white
1 cup skim milk
1 tablespoon canola oil
1 teaspoon vanilla extract
½ cup semisweet chocolate chips
1 dollop nonfat flavored yogurt (optional)
1 generous squirt whipped topping (optional)
Dark chocolate shavings (optional)

Whisk together the flours, cocoa, sugar, flaxseed, baking powder, and salt in a large bowl. Set aside.

In a medium bowl, lightly beat the egg and egg white; then add the milk, oil, and vanilla, and whisk until combined.

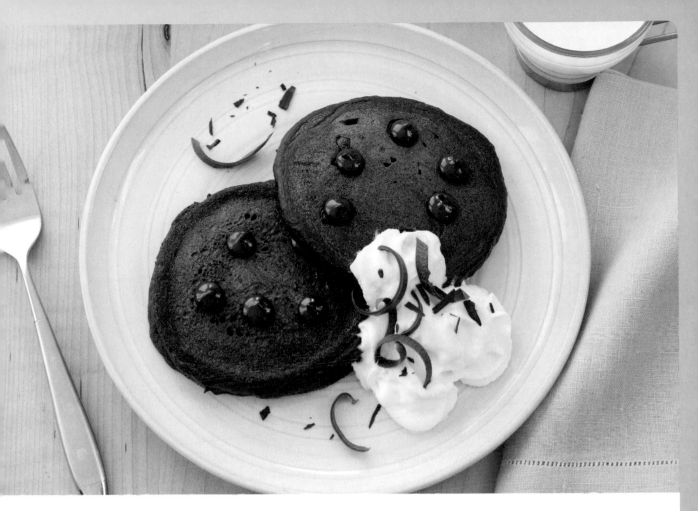

Pour the wet ingredients over the dry ingredients, and stir until the batter is just blended and no dry streaks remain.

Gently fold in the chocolate chips. Take care not to overmix, as this will cause the pancakes to be chewy. If time allows, let the batter rest for 10 minutes before cooking the pancakes.

Spray a griddle with nonstick oil spray and warm over medium-high heat.

Ladle the batter onto the griddle to form about 12 medium pancakes (use ¼ cup batter per pancake). Cook the pancakes until small bubbles form around the edges, 1 to 2 minutes. Flip the pancakes and cook until the center is cooked, about 1 minute. Recoat the skillet with nonstick oil spray between batches to prevent the pancakes from sticking.

Enjoy the pancakes plain, or add your desired toppings.

nutrition information PER SERVING OF 2 PANCAKES
275 calories ▪ 8 g protein ▪ 10.5 g total fat (6 g unsaturated, 4.5 g saturated) ▪ 32 mg cholesterol ▪ 41 g carbs ▪ 5.5 g fiber
21.5 g total sugar (2.5 g natural, 19 g added) ▪ 205 mg sodium

TASTY TWIST While these are amazing on their own, you can add all sorts of toppings to make them even more exciting. Tack on an additional 15 calories for each of the following: 2 tablespoons of nonfat yogurt, 2 tablespoons of canned whipped topping, or 1 teaspoon of dark chocolate shavings.

Junk Food

880 CALORIES

CINNAMON BUN

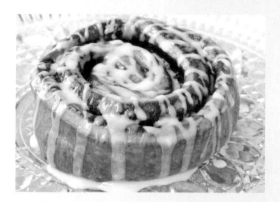

You can usually count on two things when you walk into a mall: being hit up by a kiosk salesperson peddling the latest electronic or beauty product and being hit by the smell of those delectable cinnamon buns.

I'll be honest—I love those ooey-gooey cinnamon treats as much as the next person (there's no denying they taste out of this world), but at 880 calories and 58 grams of sugar per serving, it's hard to justify the splurge. That's more calories than 16 cream-filled chocolate cookies . . . and the sugar equivalent of 29 donut holes!

Fortunately, I found a way to health-ify the sweet indulgence in my own kitchen, so you can enjoy it *whenever* you want. Delicious, diet-friendly, and you don't have to deal with mall traffic. You're welcome.

Joy Food

150 CALORIES

CINNA-YUMS
makes 8 servings

I guarantee this will soon become one of your favorite recipes—and probably the messiest page in this book. I've relied on two secret ingredients to slim down this fattening favorite: pumpkin and nonfat yogurt (please trust me on this one). Whip up a batch and you can enjoy sweet, cinnamon-y goodness anytime you're in the mood.

"BUNS"
½ cup whole-wheat flour
½ cup all-purpose flour
¾ teaspoon baking soda
¼ teaspoon kosher salt or coarse sea salt
1 tablespoon cinnamon
3 egg whites
¾ cup canned 100% pumpkin puree
¾ cup nonfat plain yogurt
2 tablespoons brown sugar
2 teaspoons vanilla extract

ICING
4 ounces light or reduced-fat cream
   cheese at room temp
¼ cup maple syrup
¼ cup pecans, toasted and roughly
   chopped (optional)
Cinnamon (optional)

To make the "buns": Whisk together the flours, baking soda, salt, and cinnamon in a large bowl until well combined. Set aside.

In a second large mixing bowl, whip the egg whites until blended. Add the pumpkin, yogurt, brown sugar, and vanilla, and whisk until combined.

Pour the wet ingredients over the dry ingredients and stir gently until just combined and smooth (no dry

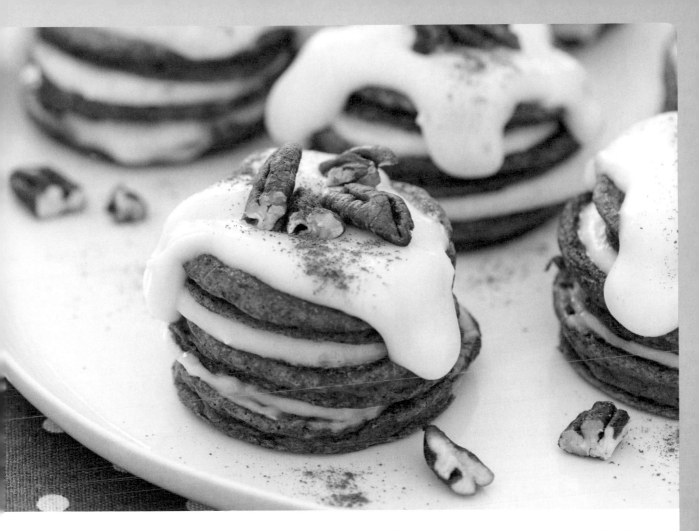

streaks should remain), taking care not to overmix. If time allows, let the batter rest for 10 minutes.

Liberally coat a large skillet or griddle with nonstick oil spray and warm over medium heat. When the pan is nice and hot, ladle about 1 tablespoon of batter onto the skillet to form a mini pancake, making a total of about 24 mini pancakes. The batter will be thick, so spread it out with the back of a spoon to make a circle. Cook until the bottom of each mini pancake is golden brown and bubbles start to form in the batter, about 2 to 3 minutes. Flip the pancakes and push down with the back of a spatula to flatten them out a little bit. This will help cook the middle. Cook until the other side is golden brown, another 2 to 3 minutes. Recoat the skillet with nonstick oil spray periodically to prevent the pancakes from sticking.

To make the icing: In a small food processor, blend together the cream cheese and maple syrup until smooth.

To serve, spread about 1 teaspoon icing on a mini pancake, and then top with another pancake. Spread 1 teaspoon of icing on top of the second pancake before adding a last pancake on top. Finally, spread about 2 teaspoons of icing on the top and garnish with 1 teaspoon chopped and toasted pecans and a sprinkling of cinnamon, if desired.

nutrition information PER SERVING OF 3 MINI PANCAKES WITH ICING ▪ 150 calories ▪ 6 g protein 3 g total fat (1.5 g unsaturated, 1.5 g saturated) 8 mg cholesterol ▪ 27 g carbs ▪ 2 g fiber ▪ 12.5 g total sugar (3 g natural, 9.5 g added) ▪ 270 mg sodium

Junk Food

FRUIT JAM

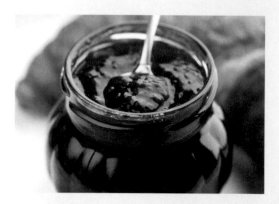

Looking to spread a little sweetness into your morning meal? While fruit-flavored jams and jellies are the perfect toppers for toast, English muffins, scones, or oatmeal, many popular brands will blast you with about 50 calories and 3 teaspoons of sugar per tablespoon (and who stops at 1 tablespoon?!).

Instead, you can try whipping up a batch of my homemade cherry-chia jam, which is so, so easy to make and will satisfy your sweet tooth with just 14 calories and only 2 grams of naturally occurring sugar per serving. That's what I call . . . sweet.

Joy Food

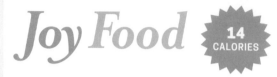

CHERRY-CHIA JAM

makes 28 servings

Chia seeds are dietary powerhouses and a plant source of omega-3 fats. I sprinkle them into everything from puddings to smoothies, and I recently discovered how to mix them with cherries to make a crave-worthy fruit jam. (They absorb liquid and create a gel-like consistency, so they work perfectly.) My family and friends are hooked and have been regularly using my healthy fruit jam on their PB&J sammies, mixing it into oatmeal and yogurt—even licking it right off the spoon.

> 2 cups pitted fresh or frozen sweet cherries
> 1 cup pineapple cubes
> 2 tablespoons chia seeds

Add the cherries and pineapple into a small saucepan. (If you're using frozen cherries, slightly thaw them first.) Cook the fruit over medium heat for about 7 minutes, continuously stirring, chopping, and mashing it with the back of a spoon to break up its skin and release the natural juices.

Remove the fruit from the heat and pick out any remaining large pineapple chunks. (Don't discard them—they're delicious mixed into oatmeal, yogurt, or cottage cheese.)

Add chia seeds to the fruit and mix well. Transfer the mixture to a mason jar with a lid and refrigerate overnight. The chia seeds will immediately start to form a gel, hence the jelly-like consistency.

This recipe makes about 1¾ cups. You can store this jam in the fridge for up to 10 days.

---

nutrition information PER 1-TABLESPOON SERVING
14 calories ▪ 0 g protein ▪ 0 g total fat (0 g unsaturated, 0 g saturated) ▪ 0 mg cholesterol ▪ 3 g carbs ▪ 1 g fiber
2 g total sugar (2 g natural, 0 g added) ▪ 0 mg sodium

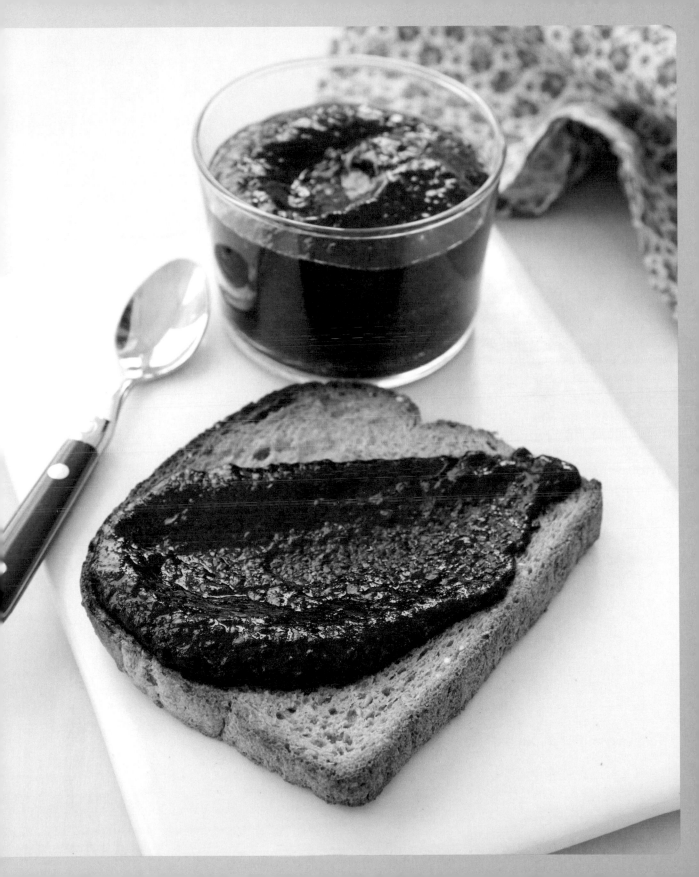

Junk Food
550 CALORIES

BAGEL WITH CREAM CHEESE AND JELLY

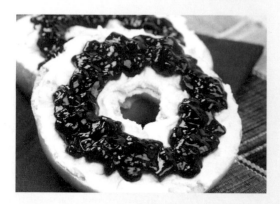

Sadly, that oversized bagel slathered with cream cheese you regularly pick up from your local deli can set you back 550 calories. One bagel is the equivalent of about five slices of white bread, and delis are notoriously generous (understatement) with the amount of cream cheese or butter they plop on. Top it off with sweetened jelly or jam and you're hit with a tsunami of refined carbs, sugar, and saturated fat.

But there's good news. You can easily make your doughy delight more diet-friendly by skipping the refined white bagels (choose whole-grain varieties when possible), scooping out the carb-and-calorie-heavy inside, and requesting a thin layer of topping rather than the standard blob. Also, opt for light or reduced-fat versions of cream cheese if that's your thing. Or . . . try my yummy Bagel with Strawberry Cream Cheese.

Joy Food
240 CALORIES

BAGEL WITH STRAWBERRY CREAM CHEESE

makes 1 serving

Add a flavorful and healthful topping to your morning bagel with this fruity cream-cheese spread, which takes just minutes to make. I encourage you to experiment with different fruits and savory seasonings until you hit upon a few favorites.

- 2 strawberries, diced
- 2 tablespoons light or reduced-fat cream cheese
- 1 whole-grain bagel, scooped, or bagel flat, bagel thin, or mini bagel

Mix strawberries into cream cheese using a spoon. Spread on scooped bagel and enjoy.

---

nutrition information PER SERVING
240 calories ▪ 9 g protein ▪ 6 g total fat (3 g unsaturated, 3 g saturated) ▪ 16 mg cholesterol ▪ 37 g carbs ▪ 3.5 g fiber 5.5 g total sugar (2 g natural, 3.5 g added) ▪ 350 g sodium

> **TASTY TWIST** Light or reduced-fat cream cheese is a great base for creating a wide variety of tasty toppers. Looking for a sweet spread? Mix it with diced ripe mango, peach, pineapple, or any other favorite fruit. Prefer savory? Mix in some chopped smoked salmon with a dash of Worcestershire sauce, a pinch of dried dill, and chopped scallions. Yum!

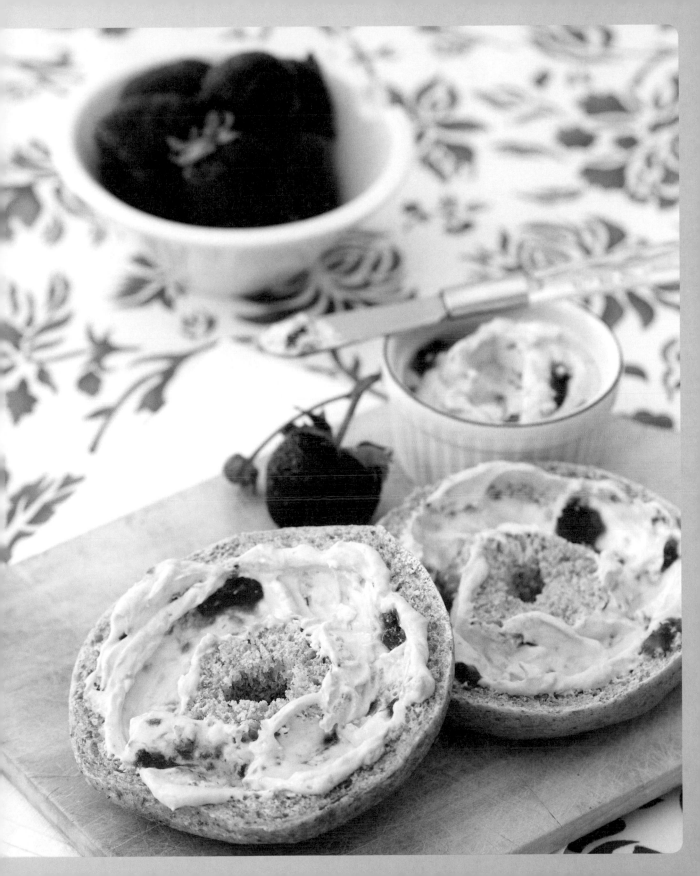

Junk Food 160 CALORIES

BUTTERED TOAST

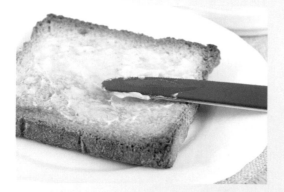

Toast topped with butter is as basic a breakfast as they come—handy when you're in a rush with barely a second to make it to the train. But let's be honest, buttered toast isn't going to earn you any nutrition points. If you're using white bread, you're getting all refined carbs (think energy crash in an hour), and the butter is a source of saturated fats (no protein, no fiber). Basically, it's a morning meal that lacks any staying power.

Make just two easy swaps (butter out, avocado in; and whole-grain bread for white) and voilà—a much better start to your day.

Joy Food 100 CALORIES

AVOCADO TOAST

makes 1 serving

Move over, butter. Toast has a new BFF: avocado. Yep, that's right. Avocado is good for more than just guacamole. It also makes a perfect spread for toast, helping to complete your breakfast with a hit of fiber and healthy fats. The lime brightens up your morning meal, while the radishes give a nice, satisfying crunch. Also, it's so much prettier than your typical toast with butter.

¼ avocado, diced
1 to 2 teaspoons lime juice
Pinch of kosher salt or coarse sea salt
Pinch of ground black pepper
1 slice reduced-calorie whole-grain bread
   (with no more than 50 calories per slice)
1 radish, thinly sliced

Mash the avocado with a fork until the texture is easily spreadable. Stir the lime juice, salt, and pepper into the avocado.

Toast the bread.

Spread the avocado mixture on the toast. Top with radish slices and enjoy.

---

nutrition information PER SERVING
100 calories ▪ 3 g protein ▪ 5.5 g total fat (4.5 g unsaturated, 1 g saturated) ▪ 0 mg cholesterol ▪ 12 g carbs ▪ 4 g fiber 1 g total sugar (1 g natural, 0 g added) ▪ 195 mg sodium

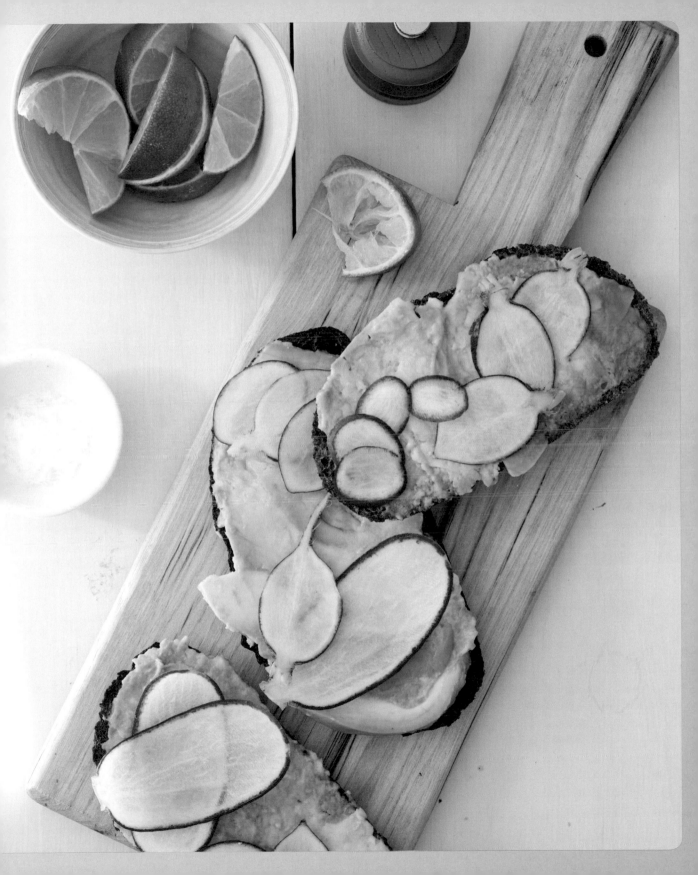

Junk Food

BREAKFAST TOASTER PASTRY

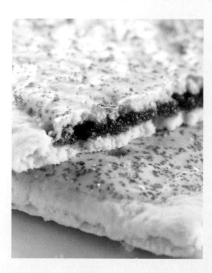

Tempted to start off your day with a toaster pastry? This might be one of the absolute worst breakfasts you could choose—it's like shooting dessert into your bloodstream first thing in the morning. These convenient eats are made with refined white flour and tons of added sugars (and, not surprisingly, almost no real fruit). A twin pack, strawberry flavored, of one of the more popular brands can flood your system with almost 8 teaspoons of added sugar (32 grams, to be exact)! That's a surefire recipe for soaring blood sugar followed by a midmorning energy crash.

If you're looking for a healthy replacement, I have a simple solution: my slim-style toaster treat. Both kids and adults will love them.

Joy Food

BREAKFAST TOASTER TREAT

makes 1 serving

Simple, sweet, and wholesome—whether you're making this as a quick breakfast or a healthy snack. The best part is that you can totally tailor the recipe based on your preferences and what ingredients you have available. I build mine with sliced strawberries or purple grapes; my older daughter, Jesse, is a fan of bananas; and my son, Cole, is all about a "fruit smorgasbord."

> 1 whole-grain pita
> 4 teaspoons natural nut butter
> 2 large strawberries, sliced

Cut a slit in the edge of the pita and slice around to create two separate pieces. Lightly toast the two halves in an oven or toaster. Spread 2 teaspoons of nut butter on each pita half and top with sliced fruit. Enjoy open faced.

---

nutrition information PER SERVING
275 calories ▪ 11 g protein ▪ 12 g total fat (10 g unsaturated, 2 g saturated) ▪ 0 mg cholesterol ▪ 35 g carbs ▪ 7 g fiber 5 g total sugar (5 g natural, 0 g added) ▪ 410 mg sodium

> **TASTY TWIST** This recipe works well with any kind of nut butter and fruit combo. Try almond butter and blueberries . . . peanut butter and sliced bananas . . . soy nut butter and halved purple grapes . . . sunflower seed butter and chopped apple . . . cashew butter and diced mango—really, anything goes!

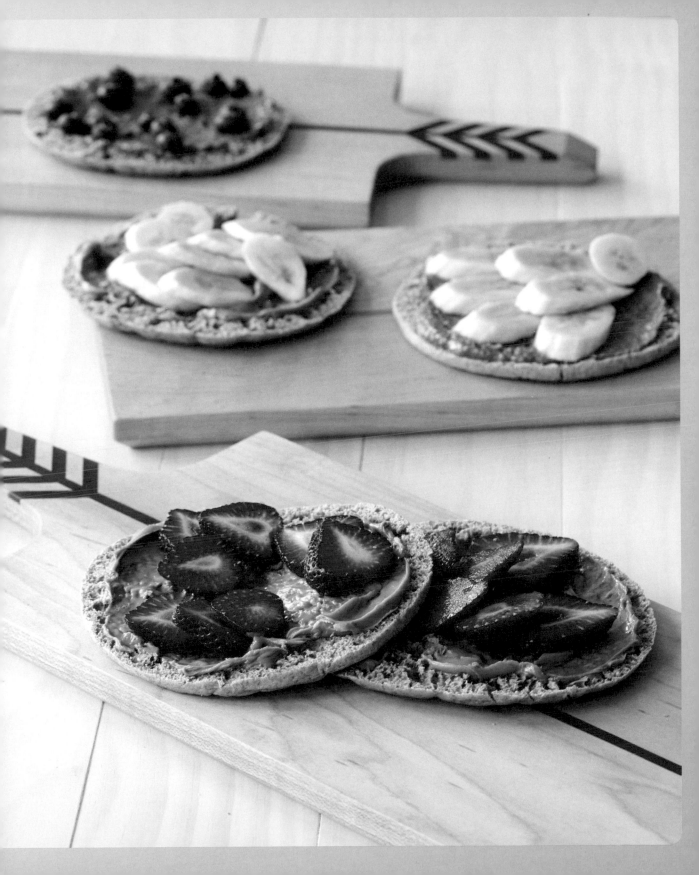

Junk Food

BLUEBERRY MUFFIN

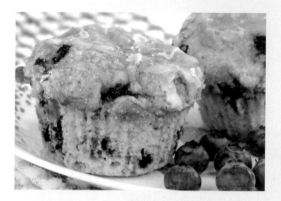

Feeling virtuous because you ordered a blueberry muffin from the coffee shop? Hate to burst your blue bubble, but even a muffin with a fruit in the title can throw your diet for a loop—it's pretty much a cupcake minus the icing. At many eateries, a blueberry muffin clocks in at about 460 calories and can flood your system with refined flour, heaps of oil or butter, and, on average, 10 teaspoons of sugar.

My homemade Banana-Blueberry Muffin is chock-full of the good stuff. Best of all, this baked treat has less than half the calories. Yes, you can—and *should*—feel virtuous after enjoying one of these nutritious gems.

Joy Food

BANANA-BLUEBERRY MUFFIN

makes 12 servings

These muffins are a triple threat: delicious, filling, and loaded with beneficial ingredients. You get a dose of protein from the chia seeds, Greek yogurt, low-fat buttermilk, and eggs, along with a shot of fiber from the oat bran, chia seeds, bananas, and blueberries. The best part? They freeze beautifully, so double up the recipe and stash them in the freezer for simple, satisfying, and slimming morning meals for weeks to come. That way, you'll only have to grab a cup of joe from the coffee shop.

 4 tablespoons nonfat plain Greek yogurt
    or fat-free sour cream
 ¼ cup low-fat buttermilk
 2 eggs
 ½ cup whole-wheat white flour
    or whole-wheat pastry flour
 1 cup ground oat bran
 1½ teaspoons baking powder
 1½ teaspoons baking soda
 ½ teaspoon salt
 4 ripe bananas
 ¼ cup brown sugar
 ¼ cup chia seeds
 1 cup fresh or frozen blueberries

Preheat the oven to 375°F.

Spray a standard muffin pan with nonstick oil spray.

In a medium bowl, whisk together the yogurt, buttermilk, and eggs.

In a second bowl, stir together the flour, oat bran, baking powder, baking soda, and salt.

In a third bowl, mash the bananas with a fork, potato masher, or your hands. Fold the brown sugar into the

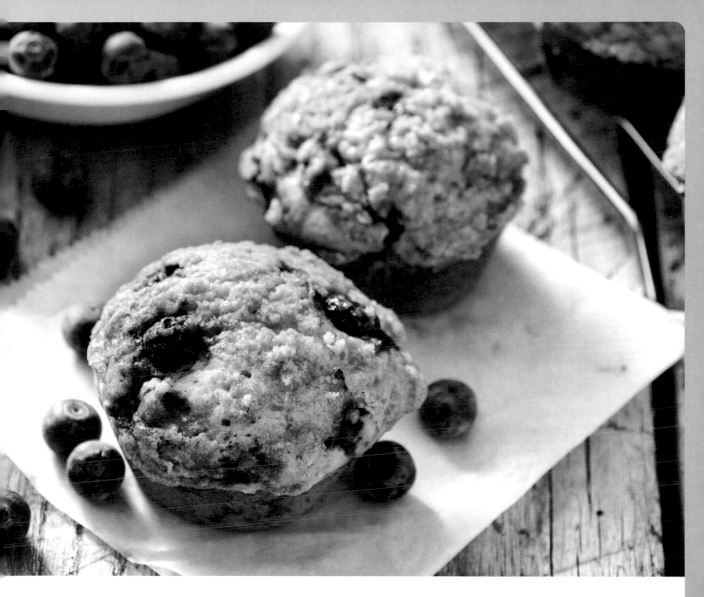

mashed banana. Add the buttermilk mixture and stir until well combined.

Sprinkle the flour mixture over the banana mixture and gently fold to combine, being careful not to overmix. Gently fold in chia seeds and blueberries.

Divide the batter evenly among 12 muffin cups.

Bake for 20 to 25 minutes, until the tops are golden brown and a toothpick inserted in the center of a muffin comes out clean. The insides will be very moist when you take the muffins out of the oven, but they will firm up once cooled.

The muffins can be frozen in an airtight container or sealed freezer bag, or individually wrapped for up to 2 months.

---

nutrition information PER SERVING
125 calories ▪ 5 g protein ▪ 1.5 g total fat (1.5 g unsaturated, 0 g saturated) ▪ 0 mg cholesterol ▪ 17 g carbs ▪ 3.5 g fiber 8 g total sugar (4 g natural, 4 g added) ▪ 137 mg sodium

Junk Food

1,090 CALORIES

FRENCH TOAST

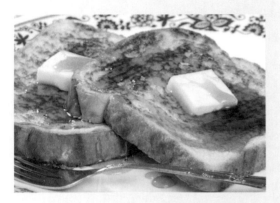

French toast is totally scrumptious, and it should be: it's thick bread dunked in an egg bath, fried in butter, then topped with even more butter and finished off with a generous sprinkling of powdered sugar and a waterfall of syrup. This combo can pack more than 1,000 calories, which means you could easily polish off more than half your daily calories at your first meal of the day. Depressing, right?

Or you could try making my fun spin on this breakfast classic and use up a mere 140 calories . . . including the syrup. Choose mine!

Joy Food

140 CALORIES

FRENCH TOAST KEBABS

makes 2 servings

This twist on French toast is fun and delicious. Grilling the peach caramelizes its natural sugars for an extra hit of sweetness, while the vanilla and cinnamon infuse some extra yumminess. Whip this up for a special weekend brunch or a regular weekday treat.

- 1 fresh peach
- 1 egg
- 1 egg white
- Dash of cinnamon
- Dash of nutmeg
- 1 teaspoon vanilla extract
- 2 slices reduced-calorie bread (with no more than 50 calories per slice)
- 2 teaspoons maple syrup
- 2 skewers

Generously coat a skillet with nonstick oil spray and warm over medium heat.

Cut the peach into 8 slices and cook them until they look slightly charred but not burned, 1 to 2 minutes, flipping halfway through. Set aside.

In a small bowl, whip the egg, egg white, cinnamon, nutmeg, and vanilla.

Cut each slice of bread into 4 small squares (8 total). Dunk and coat the bread pieces in the egg mixture, and cook on the grill or skillet until they are golden brown, about 1 minute per side.

Divide the French toast squares and peach slices between 2 skewers, alternating toast and fruit, and drizzle each kebab with 1 teaspoon of maple syrup.

---

nutrition information PER SERVING
140 calories • 8 g protein • 3 g total fat (2 g unsaturated, 1 g saturated) • 93 mg cholesterol • 20 g carbs • 2.5 g fiber 11 g total sugar (7 g natural, 4 g added) • 135 mg sodium

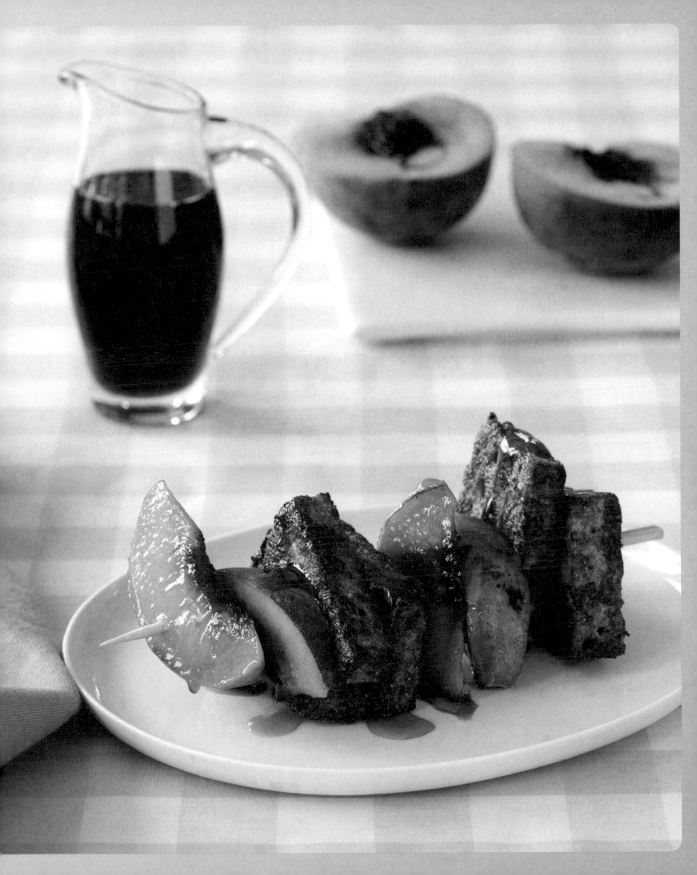

Junk Food

BACON, EGG, AND CHEESE SANDWICH

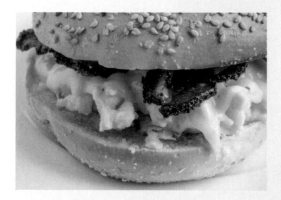

Egg sandwiches are a hot item at most delis and breakfast joints, and it's easy to understand why: you've got eggs cooked to order; topped with warm, melted cheese, crispy bacon, and ketchup; and sandwiched in an oversized doughy roll or bagel. Tasty, I know. Unfortunately, with as many as 685 calories, you're not really starting off your day on the right foot.

But here's some good news: You don't have to break up with this breakfast mainstay. I found a ridiculously simple way to slim it down. Check out my recipe.

Joy Food

BACON, EGG, AND CHEESE SANDWICH

makes 1 serving

Craving a warm and hearty morning meal that will leave you feeling focused and energized? Lean egg whites, Canadian bacon, reduced-fat cheese, and a whole-grain English muffin are the secret ingredients in this slimming breakfast sandwich. Get ready to rise and shine.

>1 whole-grain English muffin, halved
>1 slice tomato
>3 egg whites
>Ground black pepper to taste
>1 slice Canadian bacon
>One ½-ounce slice reduced-fat cheddar cheese
>Ketchup or salsa (optional)

Toast the English muffin. Top with the tomato slice.

Coat a small skillet with nonstick oil spray and warm over medium heat.

In a small bowl, whip together the egg whites and pepper. Set aside.

Add the Canadian bacon to the heated skillet and cook about 1 minute per side until it's warmed. Place bacon on top of the tomato slice.

Add the eggs to the heated skillet and scramble. Continue to build your sandwich by placing the cooked eggs on the bacon, followed by the slice of cheese. Add a squirt of ketchup or a dollop of salsa, if desired. Top the sandwich with the second half of the English muffin.

---

nutrition information PER SERVING
258 calories ▪ 27 g protein ▪ 5.5 g total fat (3.5 g unsaturated, 2 g saturated) ▪ 22 mg cholesterol ▪ 25 g carbs ▪ 3.5 g fiber 3 g total sugar (3 g natural, 0 g added) ▪ 800 mg sodium

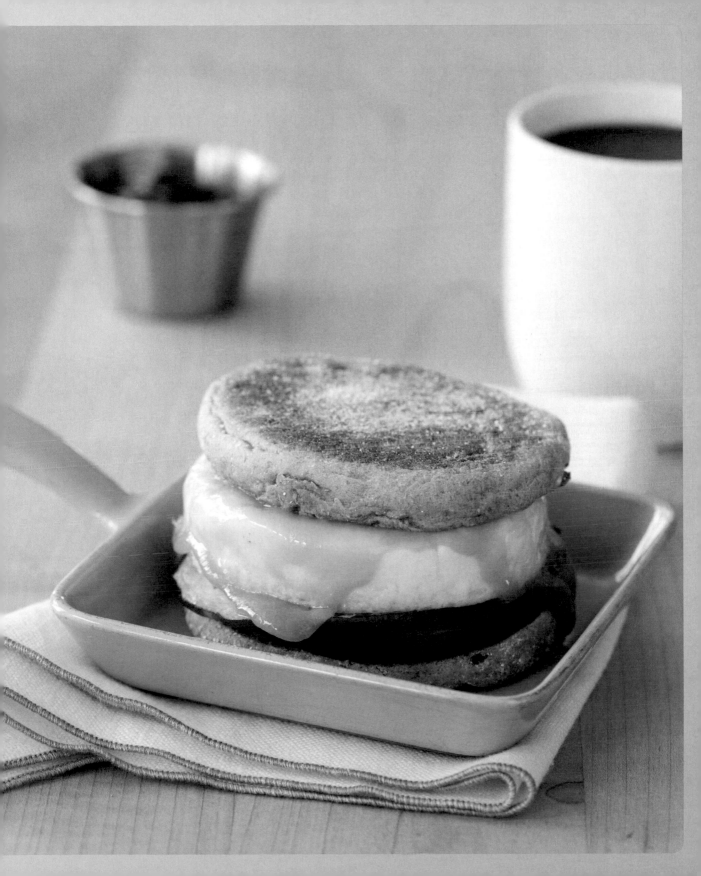

Junk Food

490 CALORIES

HAM AND CHEESE OMELET

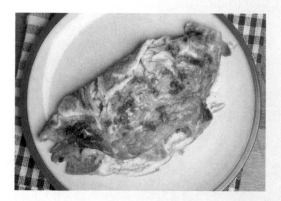

A standard three-egg ham and cheese omelet grilled in butter or oil (not including hash browns) will cost you nearly 500 calories and 42 grams of fat—that's more than 11 slices of bacon. Yikes!

But don't worry—there's no need to give up your omelet obsession. In fact, with a few DIY tweaks here and there, you can enjoy the exact same hearty flavors for a fraction of the calories. And you'll leave the breakfast table feeling energized and empowered rather than bloated and weighed down. Better-for-you breakfast is served.

Joy Food

180 CALORIES

HAM AND CHEESE OMELET

makes 1 serving

This tasty omelet is jam-packed with easy ways to cut calories without compromising its classic flavor. For instance, keep one whole egg, but replace the second and third with egg whites and bring in reduced-fat cheese in place of full-fat, and you automatically slash the numbers. Truly, it's a breakfast of champions.

> 1 egg
> 2 egg whites
> 1 ounce lean ham, diced (about 2 slices, preferably reduced sodium)
> 2 tablespoons shredded reduced-fat cheddar cheese
> Salt and pepper to taste

Liberally coat a small skillet with nonstick oil spray and warm over medium heat.

In a small bowl, beat the egg and egg whites. Set aside.

Add the ham to the heated skillet and sauté until browned, about 1 minute. Pour the eggs over the ham and allow them to cook until the bottom is set.

When the bottom of the omelet is cooked, gently flip and cook the other side.

When the eggs are no longer runny, add the cheese and fold the omelet in half, allowing the cheese to melt. To speed up melting time, cover the pan for about 30 seconds. Transfer the omelet to a plate. Season with salt and pepper.

---

nutrition information PER SERVING
180 calories ▪ 23 g protein ▪ 8.5 g total fat (5 g unsaturated, 3.5 g saturated) ▪ 210 mg cholesterol ▪ 1.5 g carbs ▪ 0 g fiber 1 g total sugar (1 g natural, 0 g added) ▪ 575 mg sodium

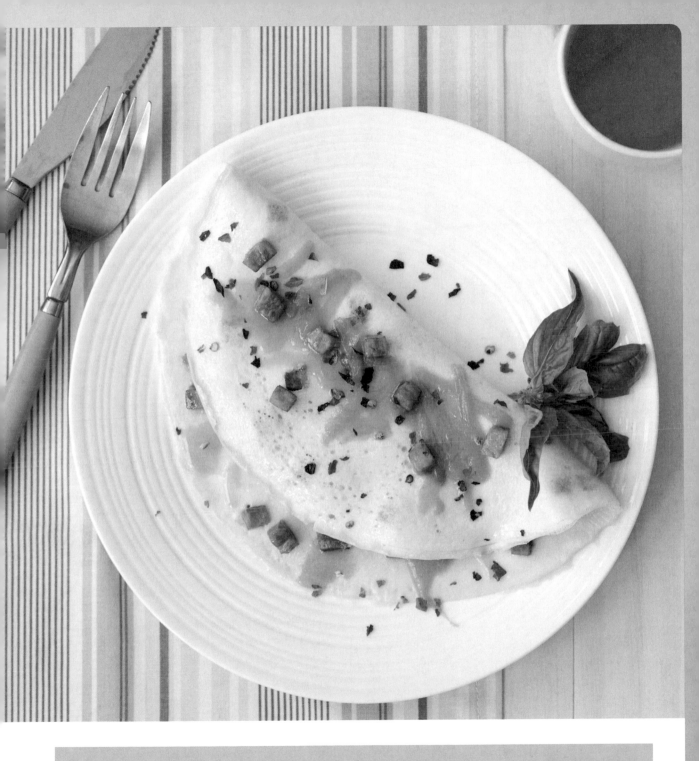

TASTY TWIST If you want more seasoning, sprinkle on some spicy red pepper flakes. Or go Italian with basil and oregano. You can also swap the ham for turkey or lean poultry sausage.

Junk Food

420 CALORIES

HOME-STYLE OATMEAL

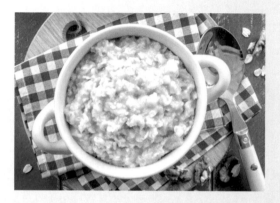

Oatmeal seems like a pretty safe bet for breakfast, right? It's a whole grain, after all. But keep in mind, it's healthful only if you prepare it with the right ingredients. If you add whole milk and excessive sugar, you could easily wind up north of 400 calories. Check this out: ½ cup of old-fashioned rolled oats (150 calories) plus 1 cup of whole milk (150 calories) plus 2 tablespoons of sugar (120 calories) puts you at 420 calories total. That's more than eight chocolate chip cookies!

I created a version that's sweet and satisfying—almost like having dessert for breakfast. But not, because it's really good for you. There's no added sugar (not even a drop), and it delivers some fiber and antioxidants thanks to the cinnamon-y apples. Grab your spoon and dig in.

Joy Food

246 CALORIES

APPLE COBBLER OATMEAL

makes 2 servings

Sweeten up this dish by opting for naturally sweet apple varieties, like Gala, Fuji, or Honeycrisp. Sauté them with some cinnamon and you've got the makings of a cozy, apple pie–like breakfast—trust me, you'll never miss the added sugar. While I prepare this with old-fashioned rolled oats, you can certainly speed up the process and save yourself some cleanup time by using instant oatmeal made in the microwave. Either way, it's a winner.

> 2 teaspoons whipped butter
> 1 apple, finely chopped with the skin on
> ½ teaspoon cinnamon
> 1 cup old-fashioned rolled oats
> 1¾ cups unsweetened vanilla almond milk
> 1 teaspoon vanilla extract

Add the butter to a skillet and place over medium heat. Once the butter has melted, add the chopped apple and cinnamon. Stir to combine and sauté until they are just cooked but still crisp, 2 to 3 minutes.

Meanwhile, combine the oats and almond milk in a medium saucepan. Bring the mixture to a boil then lower the heat to a simmer. Cook for 3 to 5 minutes or until the oatmeal reaches your desired consistency. Stir in the vanilla.

Split the oatmeal between 2 bowls and top each with half of the apple-cinnamon mixture.

---

nutrition information PER SERVING
246 calories ▪ 6 g protein ▪ 8 g total fat (6 g unsaturated, 2 g saturated) ▪ 7 mg cholesterol ▪ 39 g carbs ▪ 7 g fiber 9 g total sugar (9 g natural, 0 g added) ▪ 180 mg sodium

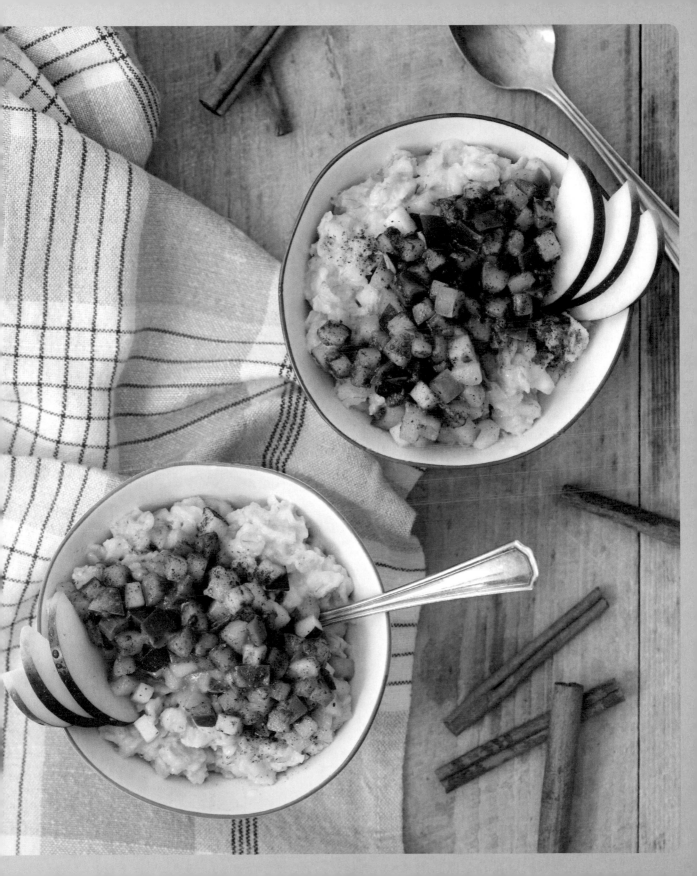

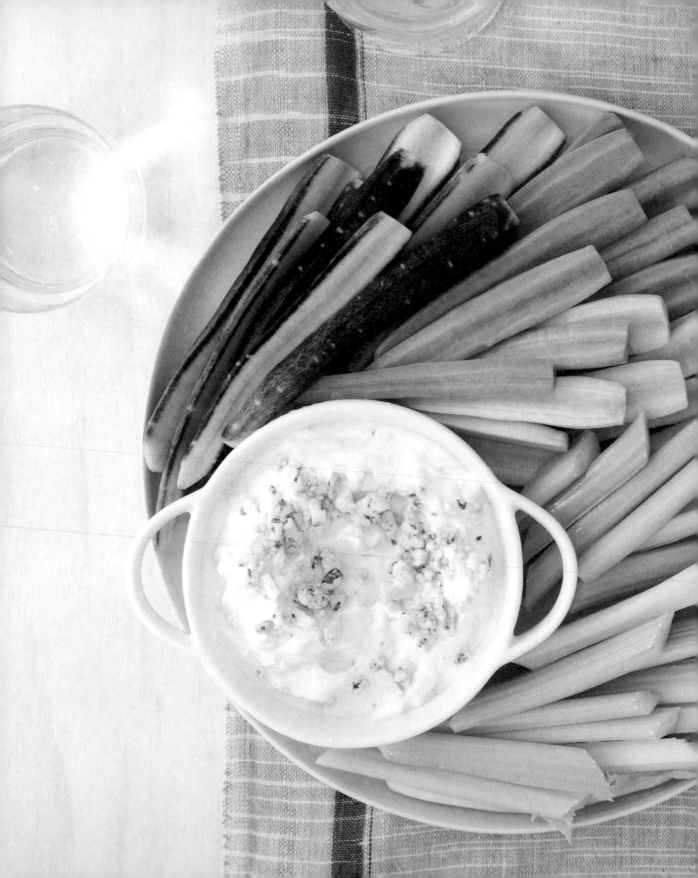

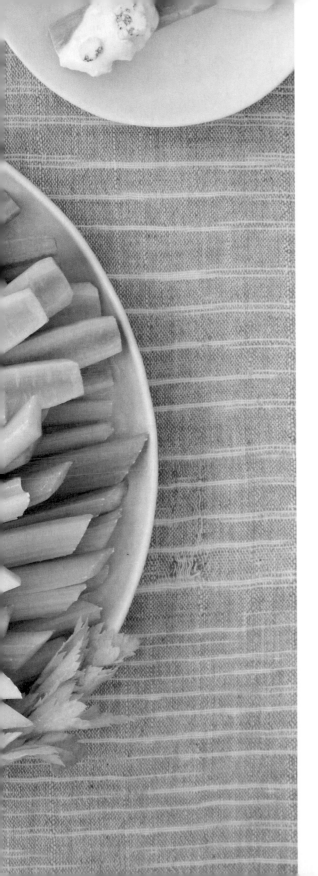

Chapter 2

DELICIOUS DIPS AND APPETIZERS

Thinking of beginning your meal with a tasty appetizer? Beware: many of these dishes go for more calories than the featured attraction. Sigh.

But if you slim down your starter using the recipes within this section, you can truly enjoy the best of both worlds. Buffalo wings with creamy blue cheese, jalapeño poppers, and spinach artichoke dip . . . even crispy chips! All of these are on the menu and can be on your plate without sticking to your arteries, thighs, and waistline.

Junk Food

110 CALORIES

JALAPEÑO POPPERS

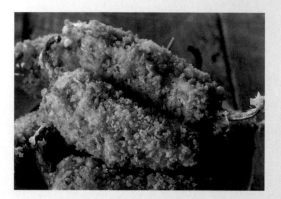

Like your appetizers hot and spicy? Me, too. But I don't like 'em deep-fried and fattening, and that's exactly what an order of breaded, fried, and cheesy jalapeño poppers is. Each decked-out pepper will sock you with 100-plus calories and a good amount of saturated fat, and because they're so addictively delicious, it's practically impossible to stop at one. Believe me, I get it.

Yet, I'm a sucker for the spicy snack—so much so that I couldn't stop experimenting in my kitchen until I had perfected a baked version that tasted just like the real McCoy. Enjoy!

Joy Food

65 CALORIES

JALAPEÑO POPPERS

makes 12 servings

I'm a huge fan of cheesy, hot and spicy jalapeño poppers. Serve this baked version when you're hosting (or attending) your next football-watching party. You'll be a shoo-in for MVP.

    3 ounces (6 tablespoons) light or
        reduced-fat cream cheese
    ¼ cup shredded reduced-fat cheddar cheese
    1 tablespoon chopped scallion (green onion)
    ⅓ cup corn, frozen and thawed or
        canned and drained well
    ⅛ teaspoon ground black pepper
    ⅛ teaspoon cayenne pepper (or paprika
        for less heat)
    6 jalapeños, halved lengthwise, seeds
        and membranes removed (for extra heat,
        keep membranes in)
    2 egg whites
    ⅓ cup whole-grain flour
    ⅔ cup seasoned whole-grain bread crumbs

Preheat the oven to 350°F. Line a baking sheet with foil and set aside.

Mix the cream cheese, cheddar, scallion, corn, black pepper, and cayenne pepper in a bowl. Spread 1 heaping tablespoon of the mixture evenly into each pepper half. Mix the egg whites in a small bowl. Bread each pepper by rolling it first in flour, then egg whites, and finally bread crumbs.

Place the peppers, cut side up, on a foil-lined baking sheet. Bake until golden, 25 to 30 minutes.

---

nutrition information PER SERVING
65 calories ▪ 3.5 g protein ▪ 2 g total fat (1 g unsaturated, 1 g saturated) ▪ 5 mg cholesterol ▪ 9 g carbs ▪ 1 g fiber 1 g total sugar (1 g natural, 0 g added) ▪ 110 mg sodium

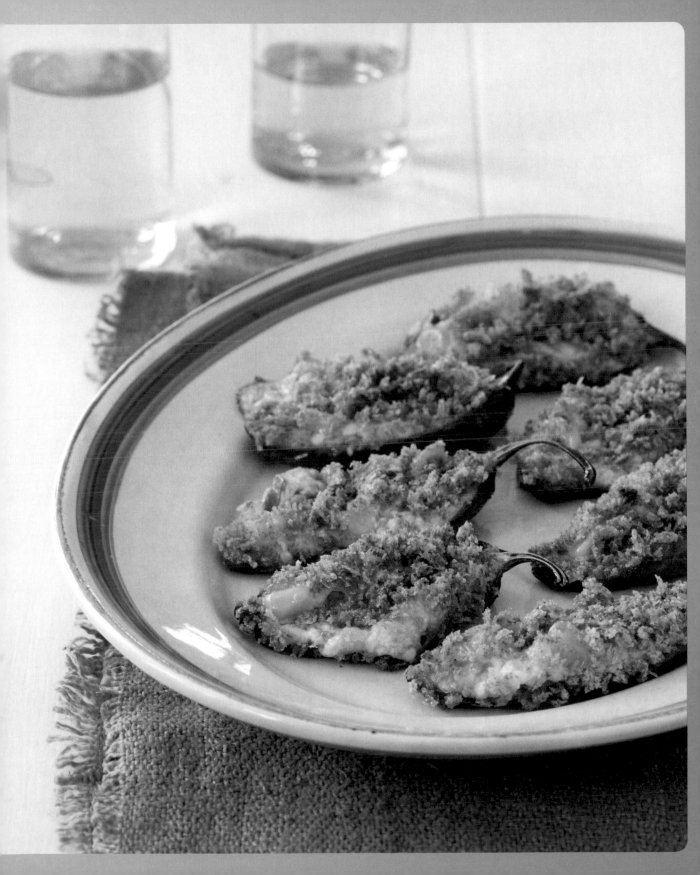

Junk Food

130 CALORIES

DEVILED EGGS

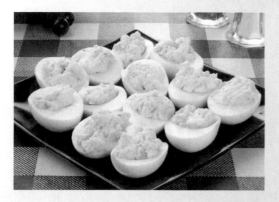

What do Easter, Mother's Day, and spring brunch all have in common? Delicious deviled eggs. The iconic finger food is known for its signature creamy middle, which is made up of egg yolk mixed with mayonnaise and other seasonings. While one egg won't do much dietary damage, it's all too easy to put away a half dozen.

I pulled a stuffing switcheroo by replacing the mayo-laden yolk mixture with hummus, so you get the same texture but with a punch of protein for a more angelic spin on the popular dish. Eggscellent.

Joy Food

40 CALORIES

ANGEL EGGS

makes 6 servings

In this flavorful version of deviled eggs, I've slashed the calories by replacing the mayonnaise-yolk center with heart-healthy hummus. The creative combination of hummus and egg whites delivers a double dose of protein, which has been shown to keep you feeling fuller for longer. Plus, this yummy rendition is perfect for parties—it's simple to put together and gives a fancy appearance thanks to a sprinkling of paprika on top.

6 hard-boiled eggs, peeled
½ cup hummus, any flavor
Paprika

Slice the eggs in half lengthwise and discard the yolks. Fill the empty center of each egg half with 2 teaspoons of hummus. Sprinkle on a dash of paprika for a pop of color.

nutrition information PER SERVING
40 calories ▪ 4.5 g protein ▪ 1 g total fat (1 g unsaturated, 0 g saturated) ▪ 0 mg cholesterol ▪ 3 g carbs ▪ 1 g fiber 0 g total sugar ▪ (0 g natural, 0 g added) ▪ 130 mg sodium

> **TASTY TWIST** If you're a heat lover like me, mix the hummus with a generous squirt of Sriracha sauce before spooning it into the hard-boiled egg whites. Or spoon plain hummus into the egg-white centers and add a small squirt of Sriracha on top of each for a pretty visual with a kick!

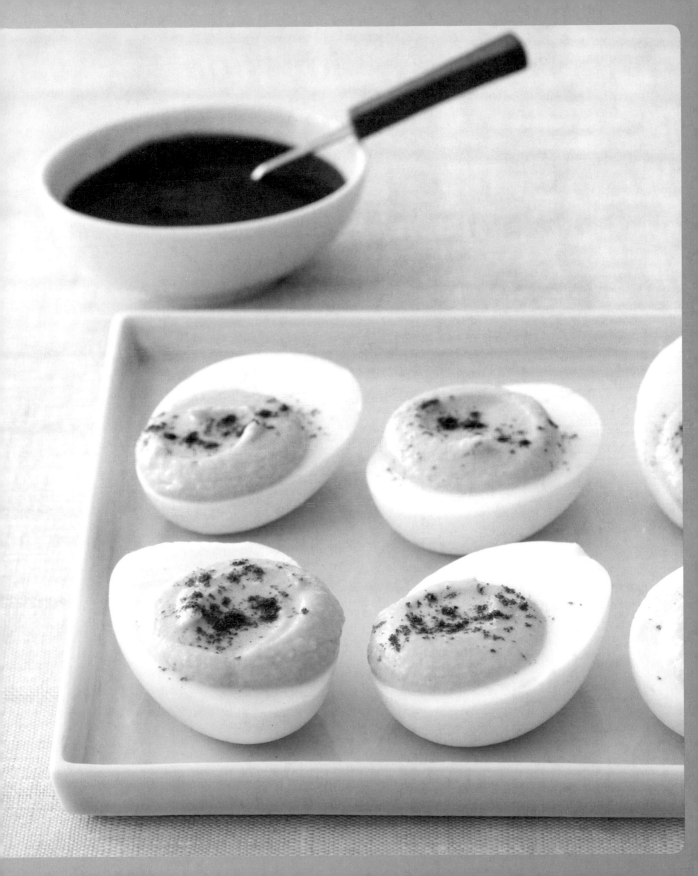

Junk Food

150 CALORIES

POTATO CHIPS

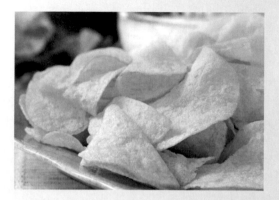

Greasy fingers aren't the only downside of digging into a great big bag of potato chips. Just one ounce (typically 15 chips) will set you back about 150 calories. And because they're incredibly addictive, you could easily put away two to three servings before you know it—so you're talking about 450 calories spent on a starchy snack food that typically leaves you thinking, *Ugh, why did I just eat that?*

A better bite: my kale chips, which give you the same salty crunch with a bunch more vitamins and minerals for only 35 calories. A word of warning—they're also incredibly addictive. But in this instance, that's a good thing.

> **CHOOSE IT TO LOSE IT** Trade in your potato chips three times a week and you'll save nearly 18,000 calories annually, which could translate to a loss of more than 5 pounds over the course of the year. (And considering that most of us eat a double portion per sitting, 5 pounds could easily turn into 10 pounds.)

Joy Food

35 CALORIES

KALE CHIPS

makes 4 servings

Easy as 1-2-3 and completely guilt-free, my super-quick Kale Chips are rich in fiber, calcium, and potassium, all key nutrients that help protect your ticker. Make a great big bowl and dig in. They are 100 percent good for you, so you can eat these chips to your heart's content!

  1 large bunch kale
  ½ teaspoon kosher or coarse sea salt

Preheat the oven to 400°F. Coat two large baking sheets with nonstick oil spray.

Trim the stem ends off the kale, and cut or tear the leaves into 2-inch pieces. Divide the kale pieces between the two baking sheets and spread them into a single, even layer. Liberally mist the kale with nonstick oil spray and lightly sprinkle them with salt. Bake for 8 to 10 minutes, or until the kale is crispy to the touch and the edges are beginning to brown.

---

nutrition information PER SERVING
35 calories ▪ 2 g protein ▪ 0.5 g total fat (0.5 unsaturated, 0 g saturated) ▪ 0 mg cholesterol ▪ 5.5 g carbs ▪ 2.5 g fiber 0 g total sugar (0 g natural, 0 g added) ▪ 165 mg sodium

> **TASTY TWIST** If you want to spice up these chips, go ahead and experiment with all sorts of seasonings like cayenne pepper, cumin, garlic . . . even curry powder.

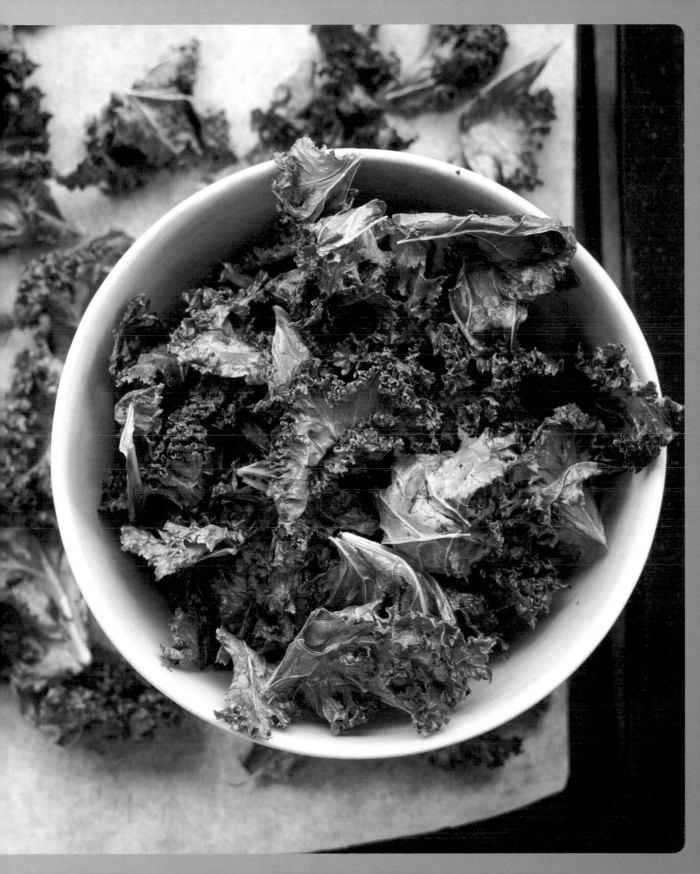

Junk Food

1,030 CALORIES

BUFFALO WINGS

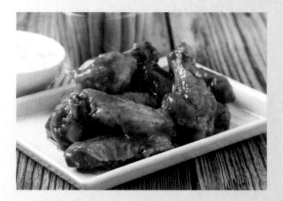

Let's face it, happy hour would be a little less happy without these yummy bites to accompany the discounted booze. After all, what goes better with a nice cold brew than spicy buffalo wings? I can't really think of anything. However, if you're watching your weight, this pair can be a dangerous duo. The wings alone can cost you 1,030 calories. Dunk 'em in a few tablespoons of bleu cheese dressing, and you're looking at 1,270. That's hard to swallow considering this is typically enjoyed as an appetizer before diving into your main food.

Host your own healthy happy hour at home by opting for lite beers and whipping up a batch of my skinny—yet just as tasty—wings. Don't be surprised if your pals try to tip you.

> **CHOOSE IT TO LOSE IT** Make this chicken wing swap once a week and you'll save yourself more than 46,000 calories annually, which could help you shed at least 13 pounds by the end of the year.

Joy Food

135/80 CALORIES

BUFFALO WINGS
makes 4 servings

I have two different health-ified recipes for Buffalo Wings, and I love them both so much that I couldn't decide which version to include, so I'm giving you the pair. Each of these recipes—one made with chicken and one made with cauliflower—gives you the delicious kick of traditional buffalo wings without all the extra junk. They work perfectly for party appetizers or if you just want to indulge in bar-like fare while watching the big game at home. And definitely serve them with my creamy Bleu Cheese Dip (page 54). Touchdown.

THE CHICKEN VERSION
¼ cup of your favorite hot sauce
½ teaspoon paprika
¼ teaspoon cayenne pepper
1 pound chicken tenders

Preheat the oven to 375°F. Coat a baking dish with nonstick oil spray and set aside.

Mix the hot sauce, paprika, and cayenne pepper in a bowl. Coat each tenderloin with sauce and set it in the baking dish, forming a single layer. Bake for 15 minutes, or until the chicken is no longer pink inside.

THE CAULIFLOWER VERSION
½ cup flour
1 teaspoon garlic powder
1 head cauliflower, chopped into bite-sized pieces
½ cup hot sauce
1 teaspoon butter or trans-fat-free buttery spread

Preheat the oven to 450°F. Coat a baking sheet with nonstick oil spray and set aside.

In a mixing bowl, combine the flour, garlic powder, and ½ cup water. Whisk until smooth. Toss in the cauliflower pieces and coat thoroughly.

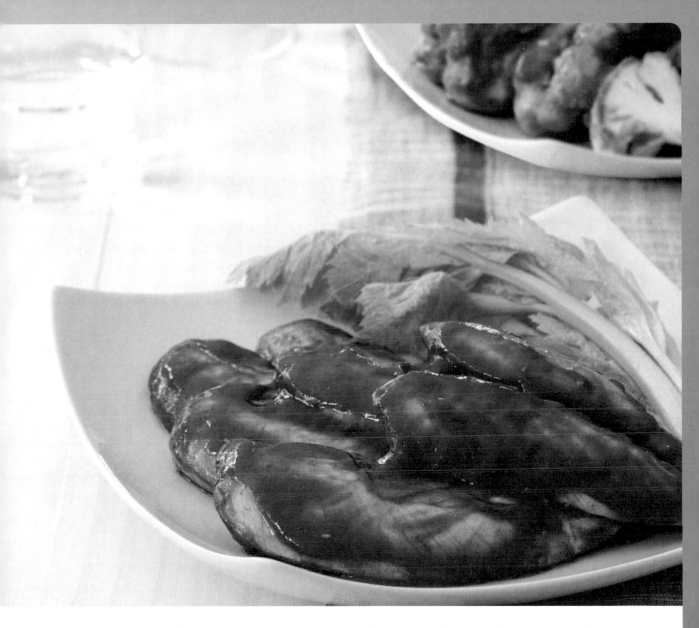

Place the battered cauliflower pieces in a single layer on the prepared baking sheet and roast for 20 minutes, turning the pieces halfway through.

A few minutes before the cauliflower is done, pour the hot sauce and butter into a large skillet and melt over medium-low heat.

When the cauliflower is done, toss it into the skillet with the hot sauce mixture, stirring to thoroughly coat it.

Place the cauliflower back on the baking sheet in a single layer and roast for an additional 25 minutes, until it becomes crispy. Serve.

nutrition information PER SERVING (CHICKEN / CAULIFLOWER) ▪ 135 calories / 80 calories ▪ 25 g protein / 3 g protein ▪ 3 g total fat (2.5 g unsaturated, 0.5 g saturated) / 1 g total fat (0.5 g unsaturated, 0.5 g saturated) ▪ 80 mg cholesterol / 0 mg cholesterol ▪ 0 g carbs / 15 g carbs ▪ 0 g fiber / 2 g fiber ▪ 0 g total sugar (0 g natural, 0 g added) / 1 g total sugar (1 g natural, 0 g added) ▪ 250 mg sodium / 200 mg sodium

Junk Food

3 g PROTEIN

CHEESE CRACKERS

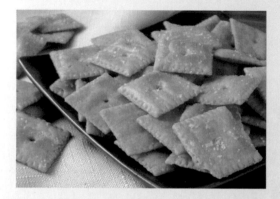

Store-bought cheese crackers may be a classic kids' favorite, but I know many adults who also have a soft spot for the crunchy, cheesy snack. In terms of calories, these aren't a bad choice (there are 150 calories per 27 crackers), but I wanted to simplify and trim down the ingredients list.

A shorter, healthier list of ingredients isn't the only perk to my DIY version. It's also super fun to make with your friends or kids. To boast for just a moment, I blind taste tested my healthy version against the original using my three kids, Jesse, Cole, and Ayden Jane, along with a bunch of their friends, and I'm proud to report that mine was the overwhelming winner!

Joy Food

15 g PROTEIN

CHEESE CRACKERS

makes 4 servings

These crackers are just as tasty as the store-bought version and require only three wholesome ingredients: cheddar cheese, whole-grain flour, and egg whites. My kids (and their friends) gave this recipe two thumbs up—after they were done licking their fingers!

6 ounces reduced-fat sharp cheddar cheese
3 egg whites
¼ cup white whole-wheat flour

In a food processor, blend the cheese and egg whites until smooth. Scrape down the sides with a spatula as needed. Add the flour and pulse a bunch of times until it all comes together like dough.

Dump the (very sticky) cheese dough onto the center of a large piece of parchment paper and cover with a second piece of parchment paper. Roll the dough into a thin layer between the papers using a rolling pin or soup can. Place the paper-covered dough in the freezer for 10 to 15 minutes to let it firm up. This will make the dough easier to work with. When the dough is nearly done firming up, preheat the oven to 300°F.

Remove the dough from the freezer and carefully peel off the top parchment paper and discard. With a sharp knife or pizza cutter, slice the chilled dough into mini squares. It's easiest to cut in a grid pattern with about 10 lines downward and then about 12 lines across. Transfer the parchment paper to a large baking sheet and bake for about 20 minutes, until the crackers are deep orange and crispy.

Place the crackers on a platter and dig in.

---

nutrition information PER SERVING OF 30 CRACKERS
150 calories ▪ 15 g protein ▪ 8 g total fat (4 g unsaturated, 4 g saturated) ▪ 25 mg cholesterol ▪ 6 g carbs ▪ 1 g fiber 0 g total sugar (0 g natural, 0 g added) ▪ 350 mg sodium

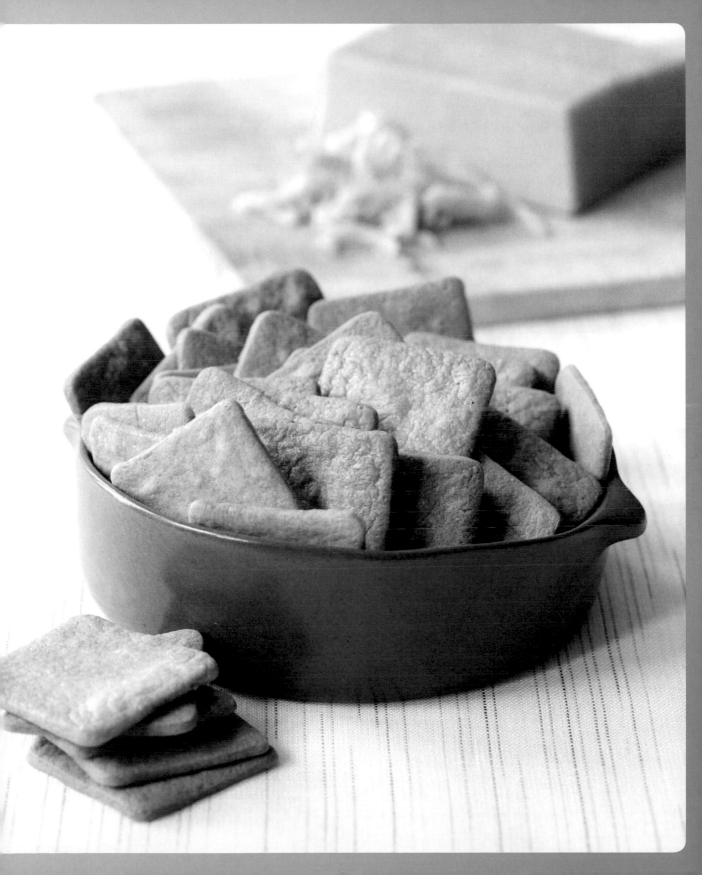

Junk Food

GUACAMOLE

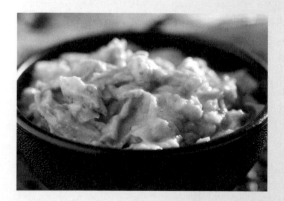

There will be no avocado admonishing here—I'm a huge fan of the superfruit (yes, it's technically a fruit). It lends a rich, creamy texture to meals and snacks, and it's a source of heart-healthy fats. But there's no denying that it's calorie dense, with about 50 calories per two tablespoons . . . and really, who stops at that teensy portion? Nobody I know. Most of us enjoy at least 4 tablespoons (that's a quarter cup) at each sitting. That's what I based my math on: ¼ cup = 100 calories. Keep in mind, that's not including the chips.

I found a figure-friendly way to enjoy the nutrient-packed dip while also giving it a flavorful twist by mixing in lower-calorie salsa. Nix the chips, add some crunchy crudités, and you're all set.

Joy Food

55 CALORIES

SALSAMOLE

makes 1 serving

Instead of enjoying plain, avocado-rich guac, blend together a dynamic duo for the same satisfaction and half the calories. The avocado lends potassium and fiber to nurture your heart. The tomato-rich salsa provides immune-boosting vitamin C, along with lycopene, an antioxidant shown to protect your skin and reduce the risk of certain cancers. It's a good time to go skinny dipping.

> 2 tablespoons salsa, any type, store-bought or homemade
> 2 tablespoons guacamole, any type, store-bought or homemade

Blend the salsa with the guacamole in a bowl.

nutrition information PER SERVING
55 calories ▪ 1 g protein ▪ 4.5 g total fat (3.5 g unsaturated, 1 g saturated) ▪ 0 mg cholesterol ▪ 4 g carbs ▪ 2 g fiber 1 g total sugar (1 g natural, 0 g added) ▪ 175 mg sodium

SERVE IT UP SLIM Enjoy with plenty of crunchy raw vegetables, including carrots, sugar snap peas, bell pepper sticks, and cherry tomatoes, for dipping. Missing the chips? Use sliced water chestnuts as your dippers—they offer up a low-carb crunch that will cost you only 40 calories per cup. You can also enjoy my Salsamole as a sandwich spread instead of mayo or as a baked-potato topper instead of sour cream and butter.

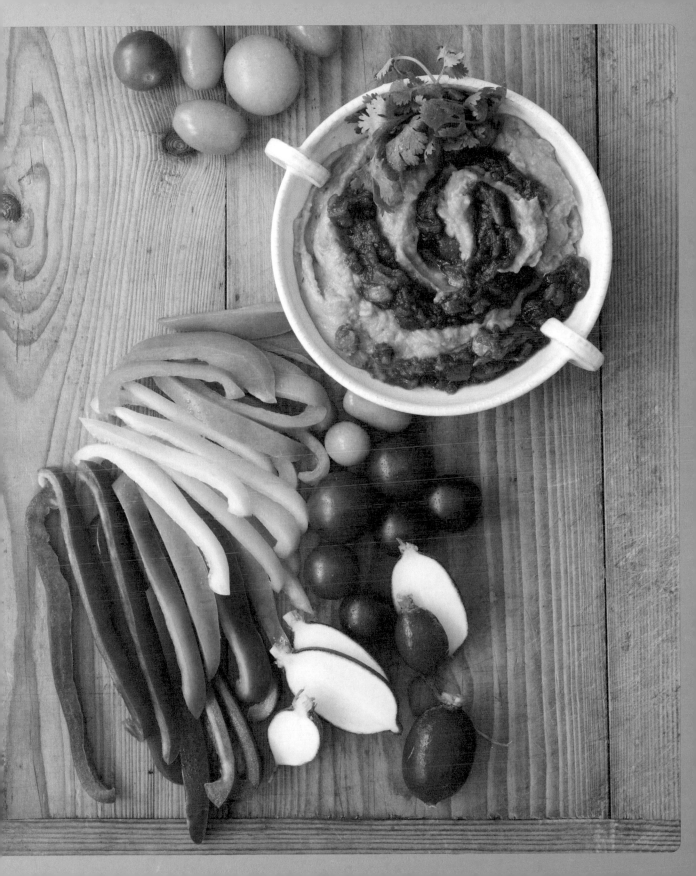

Junk Food

300 CALORIES

SPINACH ARTICHOKE DIP

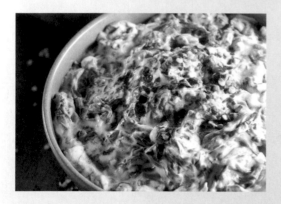

Spinach + artichokes = a healthy appetizer, right? After all, it's a dip with *double* the veggies. But those vegetables are usually drowning in cheese, sour cream, and mayonnaise. In fact, if you're ordering this dish from a popular chain restaurant as an app, you'll be scooping up about 300 calories in the best-case scenario—and more than 1,000 in the worst. Wherever you dunk, it's a dipping disaster.

My DIY dish has just 50 calories per ¼-cup serving and is a snap to prepare. Whip it up for your next get-together and watch as your guests happily dive in.

Joy Food

50 CALORIES

SPINACH ARTICHOKE DIP

makes 12 servings

This dish is a slam dunk (couldn't resist, haha). It's one of my family's favorite heart-smart appetizers and a perfect holiday party pleaser. Serve it piping hot with lots of colorful, raw veggies for delicious dipping.

One 10-ounce box frozen, chopped spinach
¾ cup low-fat mayonnaise
½ cup grated Parmesan cheese
One 14-ounce can artichoke hearts, rinsed and drained, finely chopped
2 scallions (green onions), finely chopped
½ teaspoon kosher salt or coarse sea salt (optional)

Preheat the oven to 350°F.

Microwave the frozen spinach according to package directions. Squeeze out a majority of the water with paper towels or cheesecloth. Set aside.

In a medium bowl, mix together the mayonnaise and cheese. Stir in the spinach, artichoke hearts, scallions, and salt, if desired. Mix thoroughly.

Spoon the mixture into a small casserole dish and bake for 25 minutes.

---

nutrition information PER ¼-CUP SERVING
50 calories • 3 g protein • 2 g total fat (1.5 g unsaturated, 0.5 g saturated) • 0 mg cholesterol • 5 g carbs • 2 g fiber 0 g total sugar (0 g natural, 0 g added) • 300 mg sodium

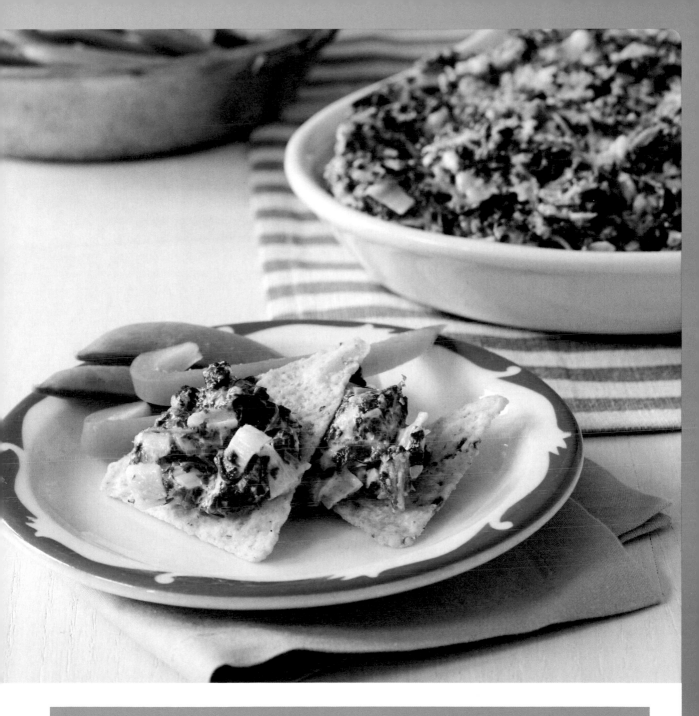

SERVE IT UP SLIM Dip into this indulgent dish with crunchy raw vegetables, including baby carrots, celery sticks, bell pepper strips, sugar snap peas, broccoli florets, and cherry tomatoes. You could also try my Spinach Artichoke Tortilla! Toast a whole-grain or low-carb tortilla under the broiler for 4 minutes, flipping after each minute (watch closely to make sure it doesn't burn). Remove the tortilla from the oven, spread ¼ cup dip evenly over the top, and enjoy for just 130 calories.

Junk Food

120 CALORIES

PESTO

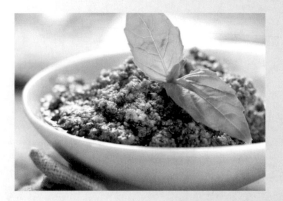

The two main ingredients in this iconic spread—basil and olive oil—are both pretty healthy. But when you add the pine nuts and cheese, the calories tend to creep up: 120 per 2 tablespoons. That being said, this is one dish that didn't need a total overhaul—just a few tweaks here and there and, *poof*, pesto perfection.

Give my version a try. I think you'll love this tasty, trimmer twist.

Joy Food

50 CALORIES

KALE PESTO

makes 8 servings

Hail to kale: I gave this recipe an extra burst of nutrition by adding in leafy green royalty. With calcium for strong bones and beta-carotene for radiant skin, kale adds an amazing dimension of flavor along with healthful antioxidants. I also use broth as a lower-calorie stand-in for the oil. The result: a delish and diet-friendly dip.

    4 cups kale
    1 cup fresh basil
    ½ cup grated Parmesan cheese
    8 cloves garlic, minced, or 2 teaspoons garlic
        powder
    ½ cup low-sodium vegetable broth
    Salt to taste
    ½ teaspoon ground black pepper

Place all the ingredients in a food processor and blend until well combined.

---

nutrition information PER 2-TABLESPOON SERVING
50 calories ▪ 4 g protein ▪ 2 g total fat (1 g unsaturated, 1 g saturated) ▪ 5 mg cholesterol ▪ 5 g carbs ▪ 1.5 g fiber 1 g total sugar (1 g natural, 0 g added) ▪ 117 mg sodium

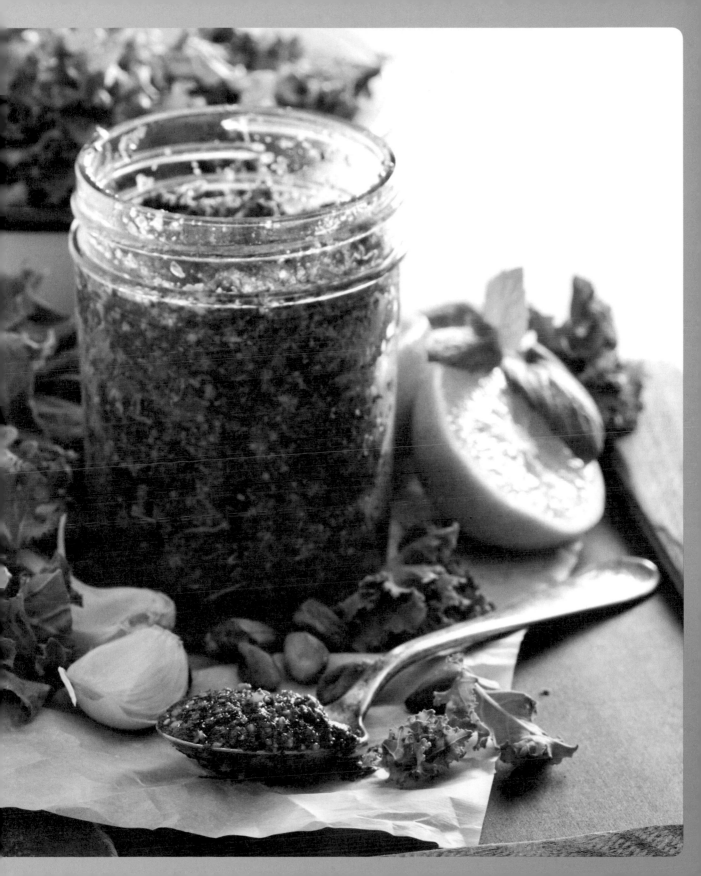

Junk Food

95 CALORIES

GARLIC SPINACH DIP

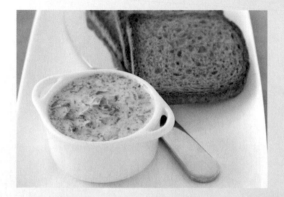

Most dips use sour cream or mayonnaise as a base, and the garlic-spinach variety is no different. In fact, many recipes combine *both* of these creamy and rich ingredients. The result: as many as 95 calories per 2-tablespoon serving—and I know many people load up a single chip with at least that much. (You know who you are . . . the chip is simply a vehicle for the dip. Busted!)

My version of this tasty condiment relies on nonfat plain Greek yogurt, which has the same smooth consistency as sour cream and mayo, but boasts a much healthier nutrition profile, so you can dip to your heart's content.

Joy Food

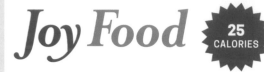

25 CALORIES

GARLIC SPINACH DIP

makes 18 servings

Dunk your veggies into this yummy spinach dip! It's made with protein-packed Greek yogurt, crunchy water chestnuts, and antioxidant-rich spinach. Best of all? It requires no baking whatsoever, so it's ready in a flash. Couple the dip with crunchy, colorful veggies or whole-grain tortilla chips, and you're ready for a tasty feast.

> One 10-ounce box frozen, chopped spinach
> One 8-ounce can water chestnuts, drained and chopped
> ½ cup grated Parmesan cheese
> ⅔ cup plain nonfat Greek yogurt
> ½ teaspoon garlic powder
> ½ teaspoon kosher salt or coarse sea salt
> ½ teaspoon ground black pepper

Thaw the spinach in the microwave and allow it to cool for 10 to 15 minutes before squeezing out a majority of the water with paper towels or cheesecloth.

Add all ingredients to food processor or blender. Process until the mixture is thick and creamy. Alternatively, you can mix by hand for a chunkier consistency.

Serve at room temperature or cover and refrigerate for later use.

---

nutrition information PER 2-TABLESPOON SERVING
25 calories ▪ 3 g protein ▪ 1 g total fat (0.5 g unsaturated, 0.5 g saturated) ▪ 0 mg cholesterol ▪ 2.5 g carbs ▪ 1 g fiber 1 g total sugar (1 g natural, 0 g added) ▪ 95 mg sodium

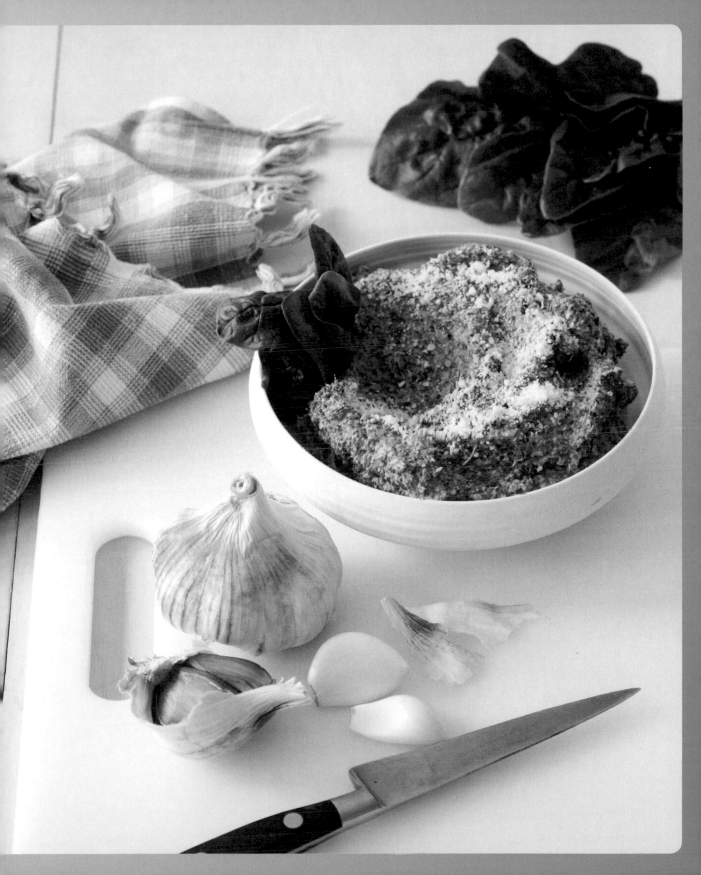

Junk Food

160 CALORIES

BLEU CHEESE DIP

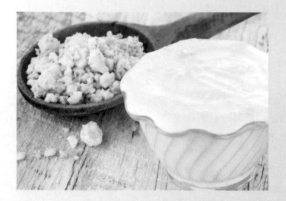

Thick and creamy bleu cheese dip goes great with just about anything, from spicy buffalo wings to crunchy corn chips to fresh crudités. What it doesn't necessarily go so well with is fabulous, form-fitting *bleu* jeans. At 160 calories per two tablespoons (that's 320 calories per quarter cup), it will leave you feeling *bleu,* all right.

Or you could try my better-for-you version, with just 35 calories. It pairs nicely with my lightened-up Buffalo Wings (page 42).

Joy Food

35 CALORIES

BLEU CHEESE DIP

makes 6 servings

I often go Greek when it comes to dips. That's because this type of yogurt is creamy, flavor neutral, packed with satiating protein, and low in calories. It's one of my favorite slimming swaps in the kitchen, and it works perfectly in this dish. Couple it with crumbled blue cheese, garlic, and onion powder, and you've got the makings of a delicious bleu cheese dip. Give it a shot.

  6 ounces nonfat plain Greek yogurt
  ¼ cup blue cheese, crumbled
  ¼ teaspoon garlic powder
  ¼ teaspoon onion powder
  Ground black pepper to taste

Combine all the ingredients in a bowl and mix until velvety smooth.

---

nutrition information PER 2-TABLESPOON SERVING
35 calories ▪ 4 g protein ▪ 1.5 g total fat (0.5 g unsaturated, 1 g saturated) ▪ 5 mg cholesterol ▪ 1 g carbs ▪ 0 g fiber 1 g total sugar (1 g natural, 0 g added) ▪ 80 mg sodium

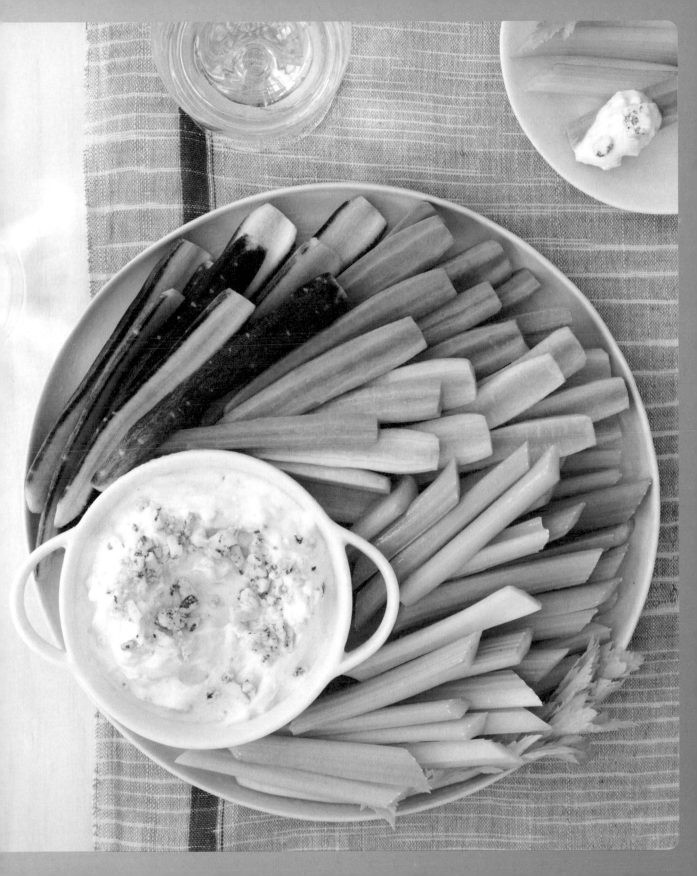

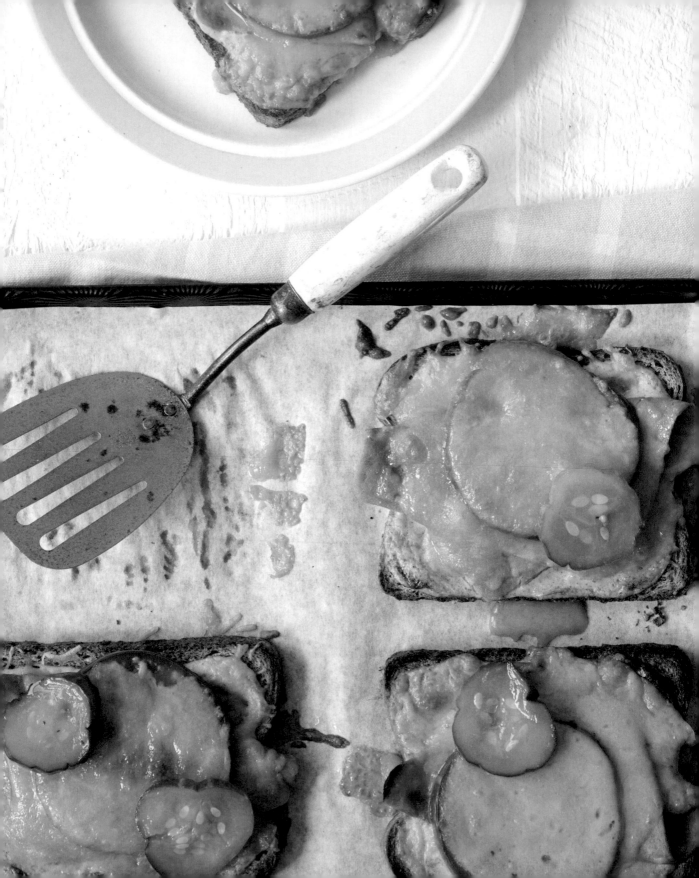

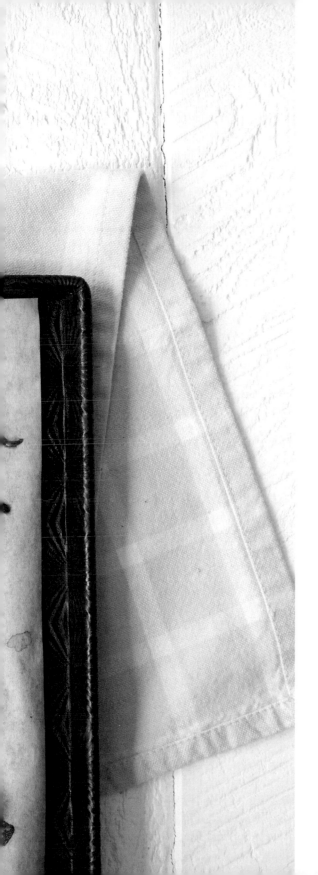

Chapter 3

SCRUMPTIOUS SOUPS AND SANDWICHES

Need to grab a quick lunch? There's something so satisfying about a cheesy tuna melt . . . or a piping-hot bowl of loaded potato soup . . . or a creamy egg salad sandwich.

Now imagine a lunch that you love actually loves you back.

In other words, after devouring a filling midday meal, you're feeling energized and on your A game, ready to take on the second half of the day.

The following pages are filled with classic lunch items that have undergone dramatic health transformations while maintaining their unique flair and delicious flavor. My BLT gets an A+ from the addition of creamy avocado. My PB&J enjoys a new slimming spin. And one of my favorite pairings—a must-try—is my Creamy Tomato Soup with Gourmet Grilled Cheese.

It's official: I'm your new lunch lady.

Junk Food

550 CALORIES

CHICKEN SALAD SANDWICH

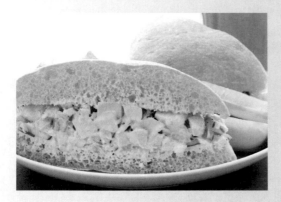

You gotta love a good chicken salad sandwich. What's *not* so lovable? Its nutrition stats. A standard chicken salad sammie can have as many as 550 calories, thanks to the puddles of regular mayo and starchy white bread.

The simplest way to trim down this tasty sandwich is to use low-fat mayonnaise instead of regular and to slim down your bread. Another alternative: try my spicy and scrumptious spin. Not into heat? Follow the recipe directions and just skip the hot stuff. Ding . . . order up.

Joy Food

360 CALORIES

FIERY CHICKEN SALAD SANDWICH

makes 1 serving

This protein-packed salad is delicious served open-faced on a whole-grain English muffin. It couldn't be any easier to make, and it works perfectly as either a midday meal or light supper. If you're trying to cut calories and carbs even further, skip the bread and enjoy it over a bed of leafy greens for just 255 calories. Is it lunchtime yet?!

1 whole-grain English muffin, halved
5 ounces cooked and diced canned or fresh chicken breast
1 tablespoon low-fat mayonnaise
2 teaspoons minced onion
1 teaspoon minced jarred or fresh red chili pepper
A few dashes of your favorite hot sauce (optional)
Lettuce leaves (optional)
Tomato slices (optional)
Onion slices (optional)
Jalapeño slices (optional)

Toast the English muffin and set aside.

In a small bowl, mash the chicken breast. Add the mayonnaise, onion, chili pepper, and hot sauce, if desired. Gently mix until well combined. Layer both halves of the English muffin with lettuce, tomato, and onion slices, if desired. Spoon the chicken salad mixture evenly on top and add a few additional dashes of hot sauce and jalapeño slices, if desired.

---

nutrition information PER SERVING
360 calories • 52 g protein • 6.5 g total fat (5.5 g unsaturated, 1 g saturated) • 164 mg cholesterol • 25.5 g carbs • 3.5 g fiber 3 g total sugar (3 g natural, 0 g added) • 420 mg sodium

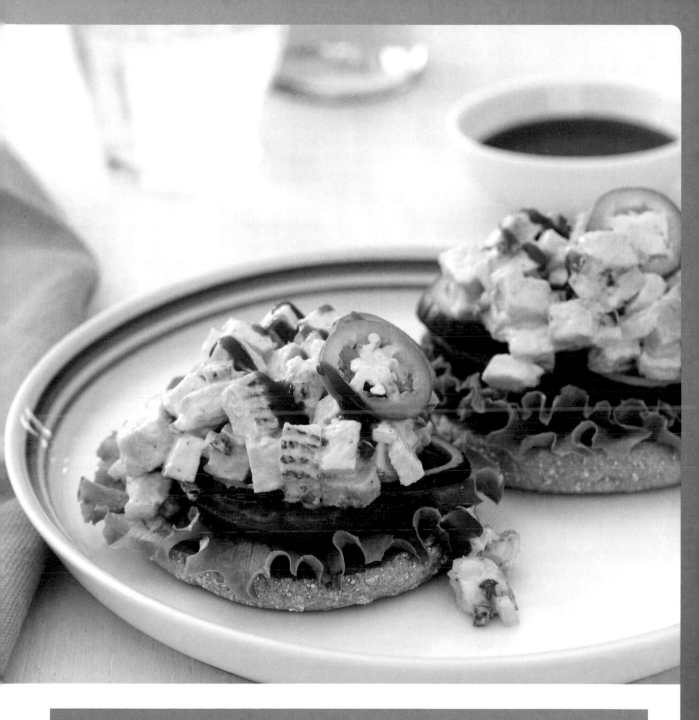

TASTY TWIST Love curry? Try my health-boosting Curry Chicken Salad for just 270 calories! Combine 5 ounces cooked chicken breast, shredded or chopped, with 1 tablespoon low-fat mayonnaise, ¼ cup green peas (or try sliced purple grapes), 1 tablespoon minced onion, 1 teaspoon curry powder, and salt and pepper to taste.

Junk Food

560 CALORIES

EGG SALAD SANDWICH

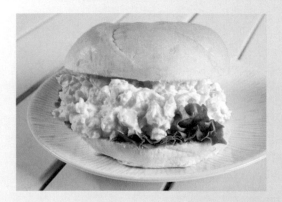

There's just something about the combo of eggs and mayo. Full of flavor and creaminess, yes, but not exactly a dieter's best friend. Plop a giant scoop of the stuff onto a starchy, white roll and you'll be gobbling down as many as 560 calories.

Fortunately, making this dish more diet-friendly doesn't require any major renovations. Here are two simple swaps you can try: switch to low-fat mayo, and instead of using whole eggs, try egg whites. This strategy works well because one white contains just 17 calories (one whole egg, on the other hand, contains 75 calories) and 4 grams of high-quality, filling protein. I used both of these tricks in my popular Parm & Pepper Egg Salad, which is delish. That's no yolk!

Joy Food

247 CALORIES

PARM & PEPPER EGG SALAD SANDWICH

makes 4 servings

I loosely translated the Italian classic *cacio e pepe* to a colorful egg white salad that pairs perfectly with peppery arugula on toasty, whole-grain bread. Aside from the wonderful flavor, you'll get a hearty hit of protein from the egg whites and immune-boosting vitamin C from the red bell pepper. Enjoy it for lunch and you'll power through the afternoon with ease.

8 slices low-calorie whole-grain bread (with no more than 50 calories per slice)
¾ cup low-fat mayonnaise
½ cup grated Parmesan cheese
½ to 1 teaspoon ground black pepper
12 hard-boiled egg whites, cooled and roughly chopped
½ red bell pepper, finely diced
2 stalks celery, finely diced
Arugula leaves

Toast the bread.

In a large mixing bowl, combine the mayonnaise, Parmesan cheese, and ½ teaspoon black pepper.

Add the chopped egg whites, bell pepper, and celery, and stir to evenly coat. Taste and add another ½ teaspoon black pepper, if desired.

Place arugula leaves on each slice of toast and divide the egg salad mixture evenly on top. Enjoy open-faced or closed. Each serving consists of 2 slices toasted bread, arugula leaves, and 1¼ cups egg salad.

nutrition information PER SERVING
247 calories ▪ 21 g protein ▪ 7.5 g total fat (5.5 g unsaturated, 2 g saturated) ▪ 11 mg cholesterol ▪ 26.5 g carbs ▪ 3.5 g fiber 5.5 g total sugar (5.5 g natural, 0 g added) ▪ 910 mg sodium

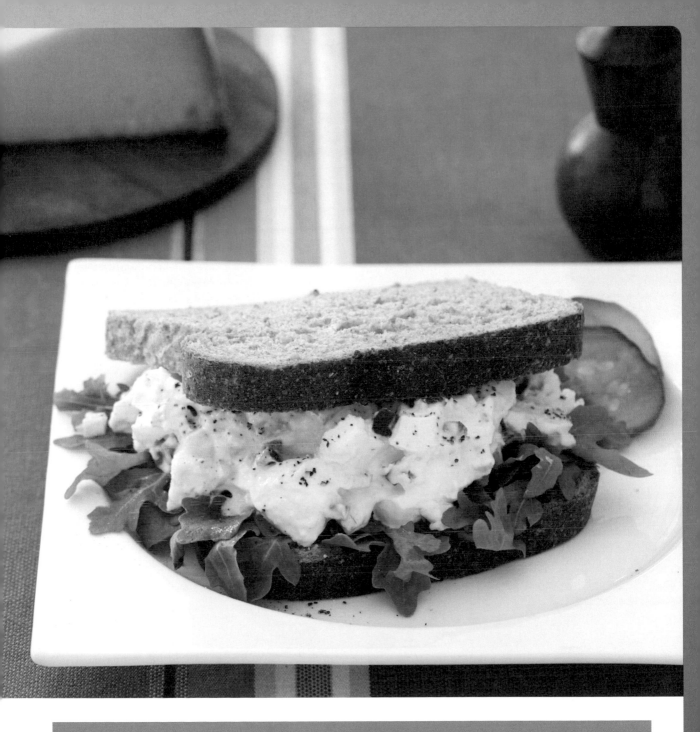

SERVE IT UP SLIM Looking to cut carbs? Skip the bread and enjoy the egg salad served in lettuce cups. Using Boston or Bibb lettuce, layer the arugula and egg salad mixture for a deliciously low-carb meal that clocks in at just 162 calories and 9 grams of carbs per serving (makes 4 portions, each 1¼ cups egg salad).

Junk Food

TUNA SALAD SANDWICH

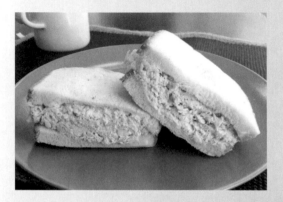

Having lunch at a diner? You don't even have to open the menu to know that they've got tuna salad . . . and it's probably fabulous. But sadly, the calorie count of this oversized, mayo-laden monstrosity is astronomical—as many as 550 calories. That's not even including the side of fries and coleslaw.

My simple spin involves using canned light tuna packed in water, which is waaaay lower in mercury than other varieties. Simply mash it with some avocado for a dose of healthy fats instead of regular mayo, and then season it with flavorful extras. It's really that simple. And yes, it's totally delish.

Joy Food

TUNA-AVOCADO SALAD SANDWICH

makes 1 serving

This mayo-free salad couldn't be any easier to throw together, and the health payoffs are pretty significant: Fewer calories and chemicals (light canned tuna is lower in mercury than white albacore), and it's packed with good-for-you protein and beneficial fats. It's also infused with antioxidant-rich produce. Presenting your new and improved brown-bag lunch.

6 ounces canned light tuna, packed in water, drained well
2 tablespoons diced avocado
2 tablespoons diced red bell pepper
1 tablespoon diced red onion
1 teaspoon chopped cilantro
¼ lime, juiced
Ground black pepper to taste
1 whole-grain hamburger roll

Scoop the tuna into a small bowl. Add the avocado, bell pepper, onion, cilantro, lime juice, and black pepper. Use a fork to combine the ingredients (you can mash the avocado to have a mayo-like texture, leave it intact in small cubes, or split up the two tablespoons and do a combination). Spoon the tuna mixture onto the roll and enjoy.

---

nutrition information PER SERVING
354 calories ▪ 47 g protein ▪ 7 g total fat (6.5 g unsaturated, 0.5 g saturated) ▪ 90 mg cholesterol ▪ 26.5 g carbs ▪ 5 g fiber 5 g total sugar (4 g natural, 1 g added) ▪ 960 mg sodium

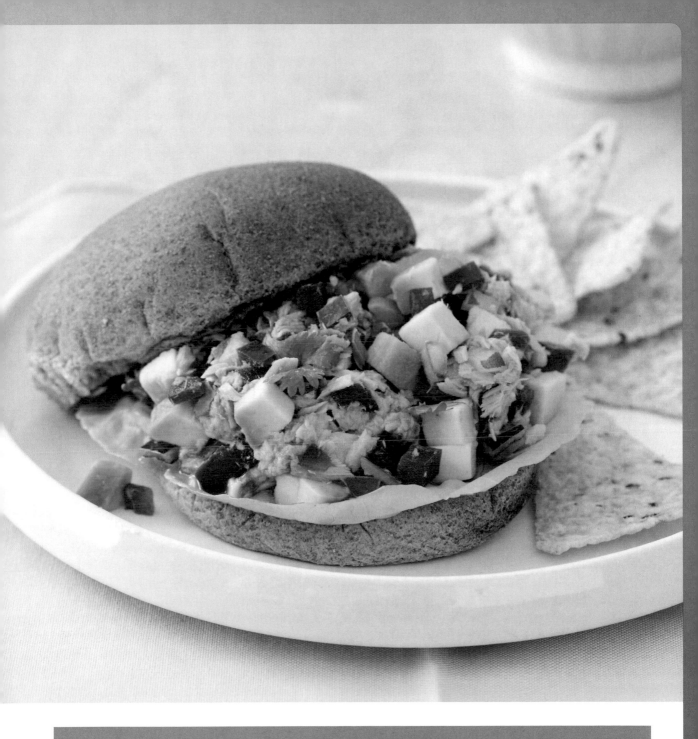

Junk Food

GRILLED CHEESE

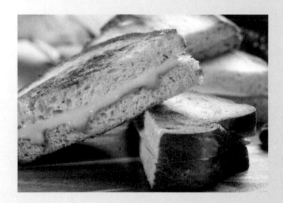

The white bread, the butter, the full-fat American cheese . . . grilled cheese is a classic that's in desperate need of a nutrition upgrade. I came up with a flavorful version using clever cauliflower "bread" for just half the calories. And don't let the "bread" directions intimidate you—it's super simple to make, and it comes together fast. Plus, the raving comments from your family (including picky kids) will have you making this slim-style rendition over and over again. In fact, one of the NBC *Today* show hosts said it was the *best* recipe she has ever tasted on the show—*boom*!

Joy Food

CAULIFLOWER GRILLED CHEESE

makes 2 servings

I came upon this cauliflower bread after experimenting in my kitchen with a number of different ingredients. I use my husband, kids, and friends as guinea pigs—usually, without telling them what I'm testing because I want them to be totally objective. (Believe me, they try to get it out of me, but I always hold strong.)

Fortunately, this grilled cheese rendition was a big hit with all of my testers, and I hope you enjoy it, too. There's certainly a lot to love: great flavor, fewer calories and carbs, and a whole lot more nutrition.

> 1 head cauliflower, cut into florets
> 3 tablespoons grated Parmesan or Romano cheese
> 1 cup shredded reduced-fat sharp cheddar cheese
> 1 egg, lightly beaten
> 1 egg white
> ¼ teaspoon kosher salt or coarse sea salt
> ¼ teaspoon ground black pepper
> 4 slices tomato

Preheat the oven to 450°F. Line a large rimmed baking sheet with parchment paper or aluminum foil and coat it with nonstick oil spray. Set aside.

In a food processor, lightly pulse the cauliflower in small batches so it resembles rice. (Small batches will prevent it from becoming pureed and mushy.)

Liberally coat a large skillet with nonstick oil spray and warm over medium-high heat. Add the cauliflower and sauté for 10 to 15 minutes to get all the moisture out (that way, the dough is not too wet). Let it cool for a few minutes.

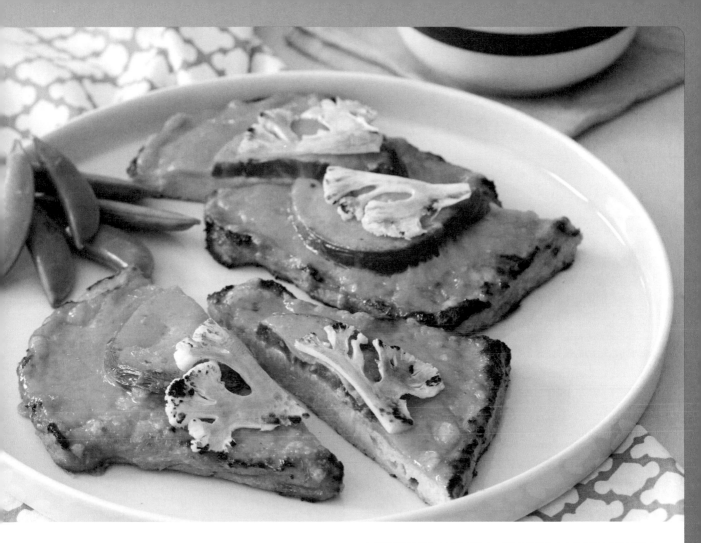

In a large bowl, combine the Parmesan cheese, ½ cup shredded cheddar cheese, egg, egg white, salt, and pepper. Add the cooled cauliflower and mix well.

Divide the cauliflower mixture into 4 equal portions and flatten into "bread slices" on the prepared baking sheet. Bake for 10 minutes. Carefully flip each slice with a spatula, and bake for another 5 minutes. Remove the baking sheet from the oven and let it cool for a few minutes.

Top each of the "bread slices" with sliced tomato and 2 tablespoons of shredded cheddar cheese. Put the baking sheet back in the oven to melt the cheese, 3 to 4 minutes. Remove the tray from the oven and let it cool for a minute. Then enjoy the grilled cheese with a knife and fork!

nutrition information PER SERVING
284 calories ▪ 27 g protein ▪ 16 g total fat (7 g unsaturated, 9 g saturated) ▪ 133 mg cholesterol ▪ 10 g carbs ▪ 3.5 g fiber 4 g total sugar (4 g natural, 0 g added) ▪ 800 mg sodium

SERVE IT UP SLIM **If you don't want to go through the effort of making cauliflower bread, you can always use other techniques to slim down your standard grilled cheese. I like these three: (1) Use low-calorie or low-carb bread, (2) opt for reduced-fat cheddar cheese, (3) enjoy open-faced for double the bites so you feel like you're getting more volume for the same amount of calories.**

Junk Food

900 CALORIES

GOURMET GRILLED CHEESE

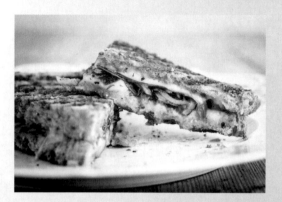

Grilled cheese sandwiches have received gourmet makeovers at many eateries. Instead of plain old white bread and classic American cheese, you'll now find out-of-the-box cheeses paired with fancy vegetables and other extravagant extras—sometimes even served with pricey wines. These more sophisticated sandwiches incorporate a lot of the same typical ingredients, like oil, butter, bread, and cheese, and then some. Which means you're going to spend even more calories than a traditional diner version. In some instances, 900-plus calories.

Want to enjoy a grown-up grilled cheese for less? Try my delicious DIY version at home. It's simple to make; scrumptious to eat; and as a bonus, delivers heaps of vitamins, minerals, and antioxidants.

Joy Food

163 CALORIES

GOURMET GRILLED CHEESE

makes 2 servings

Ready for a sophisticated, slim spin on a childhood classic? Simply use whole-grain bread and add an extra layer of nutritious goodness with caramelized onions and sautéed kale. And of course, top it off with a melty piece of cheese. Pair it with a steaming bowl of tomato soup (or my Creamy Tomato Soup on page 84) for the perfect meal on a cold day.

> ½ onion, thinly sliced
> 1 clove garlic, minced (or ¼ teaspoon garlic powder)
> 2 cups kale, thinly chopped and packed tightly
> 2 slices reduced-calorie whole-grain bread (with no more than 50 calories per slice)
> 2 slices reduced-fat pepper Jack or provolone cheese

Liberally coat a skillet with nonstick oil spray, add the onion, and sauté over medium-high heat until caramelized, 8 to 10 minutes. Stir frequently to avoid burning.

Add the garlic and kale to the skillet and cook, stirring frequently, until kale has wilted significantly, about 2 minutes.

Preheat the broiler and toast the bread.

Divide the kale mixture evenly between the two slices of toast. Add a slice of cheese on top of the veggie mixture and pop under the broiler until the cheese is melted, 1 to 2 minutes.

Cut each slice in half and enjoy open-faced.

---

nutrition information PER SERVING
163 calories ▪ 12.5 g protein ▪ 6 g total fat (3 g unsaturated, 3 g saturated) ▪ 16 mg cholesterol ▪ 18 g carbs ▪ 4 g fiber 3 g total sugar (2 g natural, 1 g added) ▪ 274 mg sodium

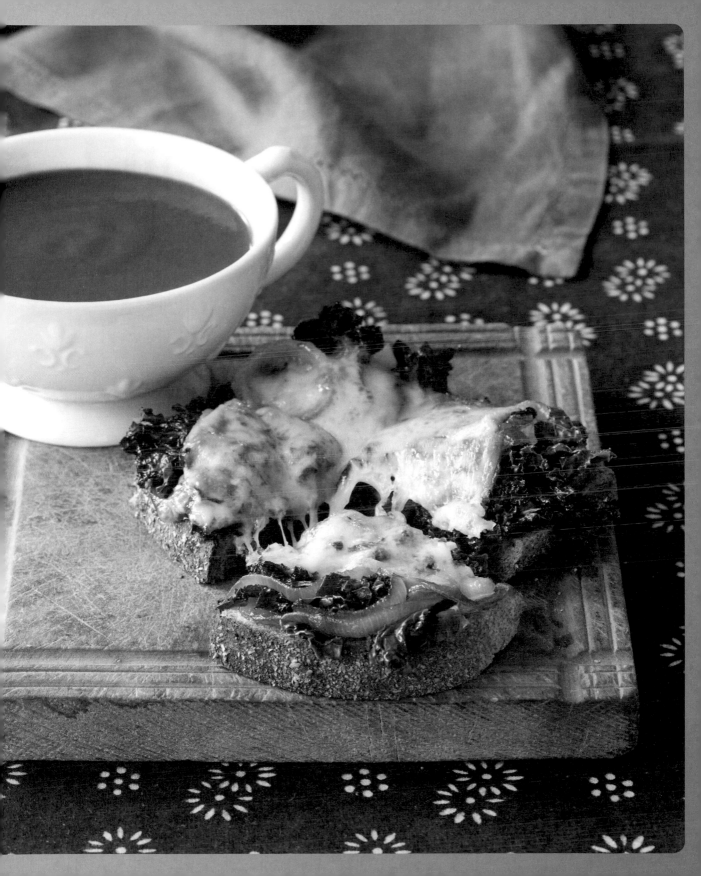

Junk Food

790 CALORIES

TUNA MELT

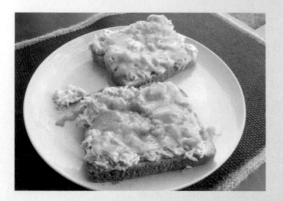

Diner versions of this popular pick consist of refined white bread grilled in butter, tuna mashed with full-fat mayo, and lots of cheese. Confession: I've eaten my fair share prior to my nutrition career—this was one of my favorite picks at the Blauvelt Coach Diner when I was a teen. Fast-forward several years, and I now know one of these sammies could set you back 790 calories. Whoa, that's certainly a lot to sink into a sandwich.

But good news: I've given this dish a dramatic makeover that is low in calories but fat on flavor.

Joy Food

365 CALORIES

TUNA MELT

makes 1 serving

Considering that the classic version of this tasty sandwich was a personal childhood favorite, it was only a matter of time before I tackled the transformation. Now I can take a slim stroll down memory lane whenever I want. My all-star recipe incorporates fiber-rich whole-grain bread, canned light tuna (canned albacore white tuna is high in mercury) mixed with low-fat mayo, and is topped with the signature bubbly, melted cheese. Serve it open-faced for twice the volume and dig in.

- 2 pieces reduced-calorie, whole-grain bread (with no more than 50 calories per slice)
- 6 ounces canned light tuna, packed in water, drained well
- 2 teaspoons low-fat mayonnaise
- 2 teaspoons minced onion
- 4 tomato slices
- 4 onion slices
- Pickles (optional)
- 4 tablespoons reduced-fat shredded cheese, any variety

Preheat the broiler and lightly toast the bread.

Mash the tuna with the mayonnaise and onion.

Spread the tuna mixture evenly over each slice of bread and top each with 2 tomato slices, 2 onion slices, pickles, if desired, and 2 tablespoons cheese. Place back under the broiler until the cheese is hot and bubbly. Enjoy open-faced.

---

nutrition information PER SERVING
365 calories ▪ 46 g protein ▪ 6.5 g total fat (3.5 g unsaturated, 3 g saturated) ▪ 105 mg cholesterol ▪ 28 g carbs ▪ 5 g fiber 5 g total sugar (5 g natural, 0 g added) ▪ 950 mg sodium

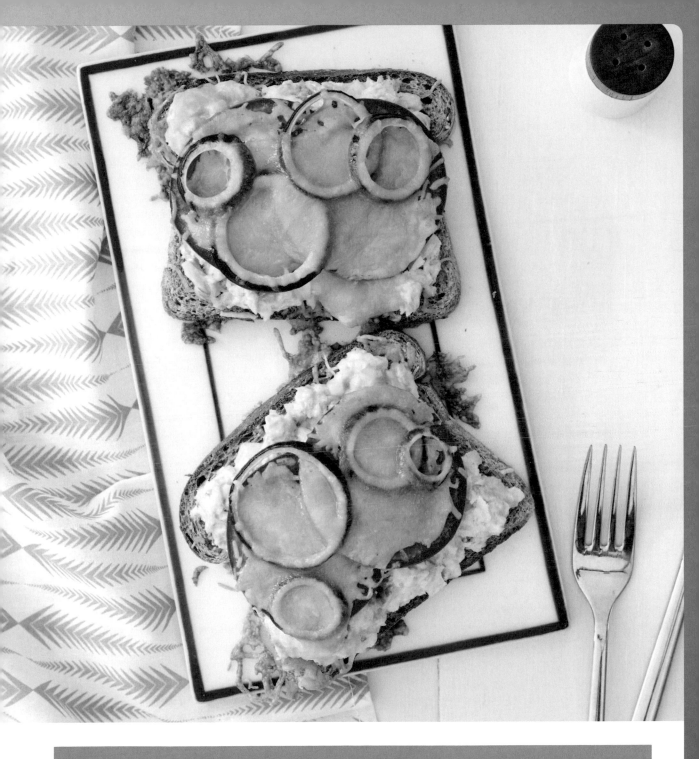

TASTY TWIST Feel free to mix your favorite seasonings with the tuna for some extra pizzazz: dill, black pepper, red pepper flakes . . . anything goes.

Junk Food

630 CALORIES

SLOPPY JOES

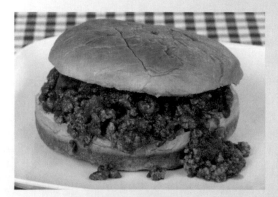

If you grew up eating sloppy joes, then you already know this dish makes a delicious mess. But take a peek at the nutrition label of some store-bought versions, and you may be surprised to see a long list of ingredients, which often includes corn syrup. Add the ground beef and bread, and this childhood favorite can set you back a not-so-neat 630 calories.

Forget sloppy joes from a can. I've roconstructed this yummy, comforting treat and turned it into a wholesome meal.

Joy Food

295 CALORIES

SIMPLE SLOPPY JOES

makes 6 servings

Get your hands dirty with this easy-peasy sloppy joe recipe. It's quick, tasty, and packed with protein. I typically whip it up for dinner when I've had a hectic day and don't feel like fussing. At Bistro Bauer, I serve it open-faced so we can enjoy two "sandwiches" for the price of one.

> ½ onion, chopped
> 1¼ pounds ground turkey (at least 90 percent lean)
> ½ cup ketchup
> 1 tablespoon brown sugar
> 1 teaspoon garlic powder
> 1 teaspoon mustard
> Ground black pepper to taste
> 6 whole-grain buns or English muffins, split

Coat a large skillet with nonstick oil spray and warm over medium-high heat. Add the onion and sauté until softened and browned, about 5 minutes. If the onion starts to stick, mist with additional oil spray.

Add the ground turkey to the skillet and cook, breaking apart the meat and mixing occasionally, until the meat is cooked and browned, about 5 minutes. Drain visible fat from the pan.

Add the ketchup, brown sugar, garlic, mustard, and pepper to the skillet and mix thoroughly. Cook for an additional 3 minutes.

Toast the buns while the meat is cooking.

Divide the mixture between 12 toasted bun halves, garnish with optional greens, and serve open-faced.

nutrition information PER SERVING OF 2 HALVES
295 calories ▪ 24 g protein ▪ 9 g total fat (7 g unsaturated, 2 g saturated) ▪ 70 mg cholesterol ▪ 31 g carbs ▪ 4 g fiber 8 g total sugar (4 g natural, 4 g added) ▪ 500 mg sodium

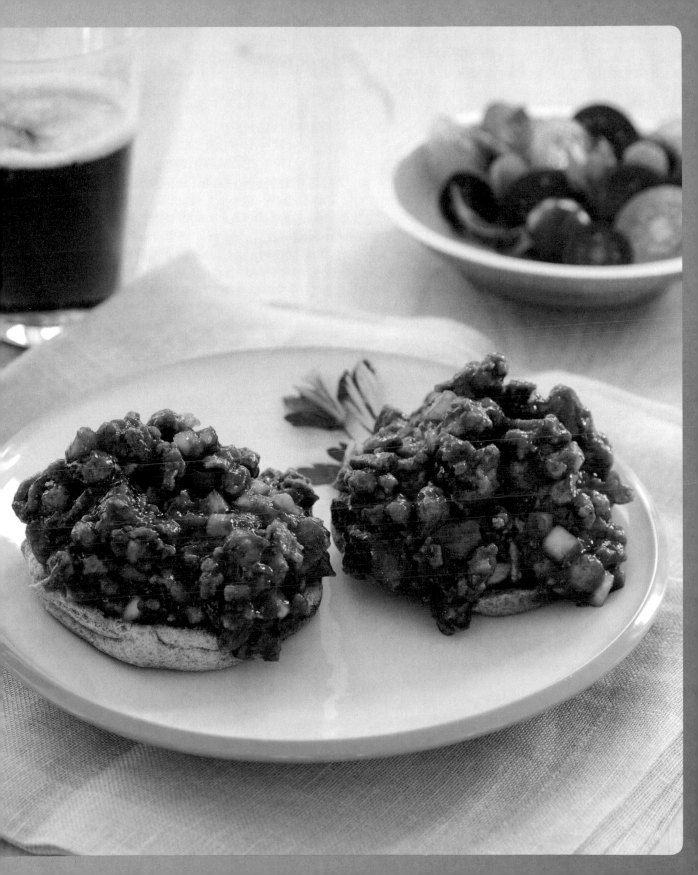

Junk Food

580 CALORIES

BLT

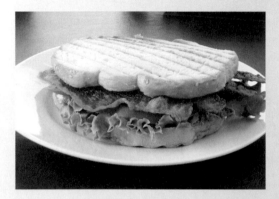

Your standard BLT doesn't sound so bad, right? But other than a slice or two of tomato and lettuce, this sandwich is devoid of any real nutrients, and yet it will cost you 580 calories. It's sort of like spending a whole lot of money in a store and walking out empty-handed.

If you're a bacon lover, my new and improved, slimmed-down creation is definitely for you.

CHOOSE IT TO LOSE IT
Make this sandwich switch twice a week and you'll cut out more than 35,000 calories annually, which could translate to a loss of 10 pounds in a year's time.

Joy Food

240 CALORIES

BLT: A+

makes 1 serving

My better-for-you BLT has fewer calories than the classic and scores an A+ for A-vocado. By using creamy avocado in place of mayo, this sandwich delivers more nutrients, including potassium, B vitamins, fiber, and folate, to name just a few. I also use whole-grain bread and swap out traditional fatty bacon for leaner turkey bacon. Of course, the lettuce and tomato retain their invite to the party.

> 2 slices reduced-calorie whole-grain bread
>   (with no more than 50 calories per slice)
> ¼ avocado, sliced
> 2 slices turkey bacon
> 2 to 4 lettuce leaves
> 2 to 3 slices tomato
> Salt and pepper to taste

Toast the bread.

Mash the avocado with a fork and spread a thin layer on each slice.

Prepare the turkey bacon as directed on the package, and drain thoroughly on paper towels.

Layer 1 slice of toast with the lettuce, tomato, and cooked turkey bacon. Add salt and pepper to taste. Top with the second slice of toast. (Alternatively, you can layer each half with the fixings and enjoy open-faced.)

---

nutrition information PER SERVING
240 calories ▪ 10 g protein ▪ 11 g total fat (8 g unsaturated, 3 g saturated) ▪ 30 mg cholesterol ▪ 22 g carbs ▪ 6 g fiber 3 g total sugar (3 g natural, 0 g added) ▪ 512 mg sodium

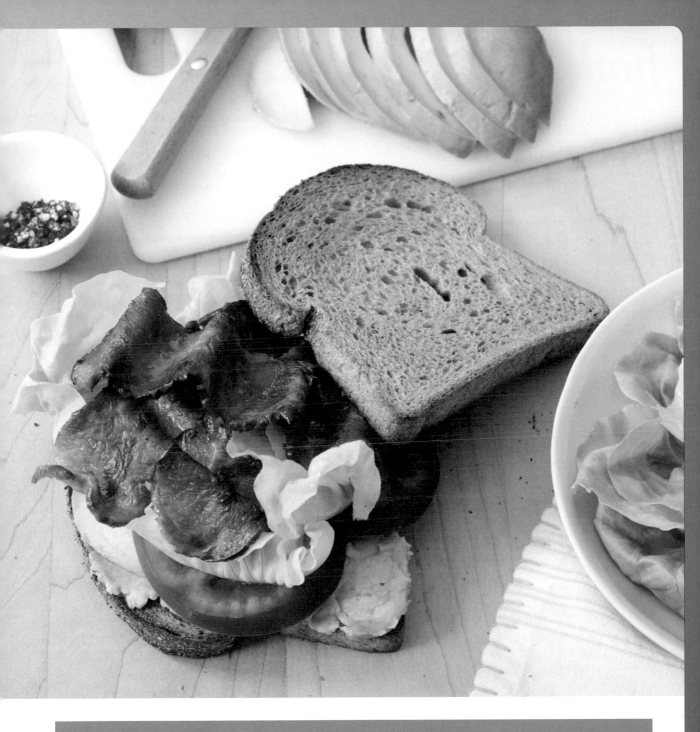

TASTY TWIST Instead of mashed avocado, use 2 tablespoons of low-fat mayonnaise, hummus, nonfat plain Greek yogurt, or even try flavorful bean spread. Looking to save even more calories and carbs? Feel free to bypass the bread and wrap your bacon, tomato, and avocado slices in lettuce. For just 170 calories, this slimming serving suggestion makes a perfect afternoon snack.

Junk Food

630 CALORIES

HAM AND CHEESE SANDWICH

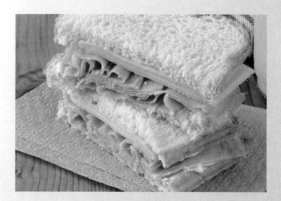

Order a ham and cheese from your favorite sandwich shop, and you'll be chowing down on starchy bread, salty ham, full-fat cheese, and plenty of mayo. All together, this sammie adds up to about 630 calories—not the best way to energize your afternoon.

My new and improved alternative is lighter on your wallet and your waistline.

Joy Food

280 CALORIES

HAM AND CHEESE SANDWICH

makes 1 serving

I'm happy to introduce my super-duper, warm and delicious ham and cheese sammie for when you're craving a cozy lunch at home. If you need a brown-bag version for work, skip the broiler, swap the shredded cheese for two thin slices, and use the same ingredients to build a quick and totable sandwich. No matter which way you prepare it—hot or cold—it's simple and satisfying.

> 2 slices reduced-calorie whole-grain bread (with no more than 50 calories per slice)
> 1 tablespoon spicy brown mustard
> 1 tablespoon low-fat mayonnaise
> 2 ounces lean, reduced-sodium deli ham (about 4 slices)
> 4 slices tomato
> 4 tablespoons shredded reduced-fat cheese, any variety
> Pickle rounds (optional)

Preheat the broiler, and toast the bread.

Mix the mustard and mayonnaise.

Spread each slice of bread with half the mustard-mayonnaise mixture. Top each half with the ham, tomato, and cheese.

Place the pieces under the broiler until the cheese is hot and bubbly.

Cut each slice in half, garnish with pickle rounds, if desired, and enjoy open-faced.

---

nutrition information PER SERVING
280 calories ▪ 24 g protein ▪ 9 g total fat (5 g unsaturated, 4 g saturated) ▪ 54 mg cholesterol ▪ 27 g carbs ▪ 4 g fiber 3 g total sugar (3 g natural, 0 g added) ▪ 950 mg sodium

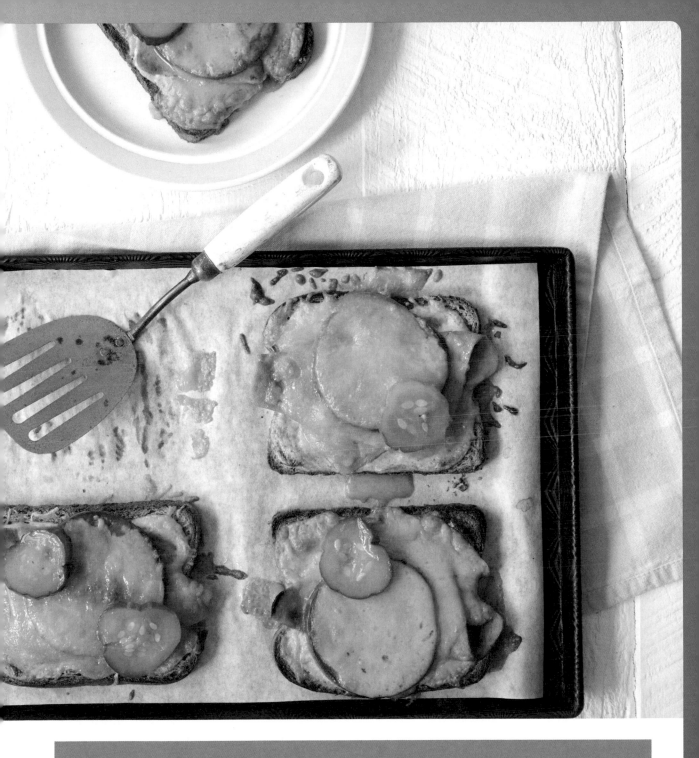

TASTY TWIST Swap the bread for a whole-grain or low-carb tortilla and layer everything on top (use 2 thin slices of cheese instead of shredded), roll it up, and slice into 4 to 5 pinwheels.

Junk Food

410 CALORIES

PB&J

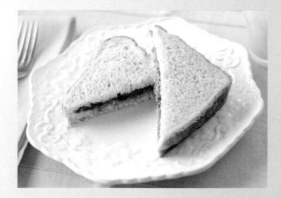

It's no secret that peanut butter and jelly make a perfect pair, especially in sandwich form. And while a PB&J sammie is definitely simple and oh-so-easy to put together, there's room for improvement. Exhibit A: PB&Js have about 410 calories and 18 grams of sugar (that's about 4 teaspoons of sugar, the equivalent of 25 jelly beans).

My version of this kiddie classic (that grown-ups can eat and enjoy, too!), is still just as nutty, gooey, and richly delicious. Make it once, and you'll make it a thousand times. Best part? It's so simple. You'll see.

Joy Food

300 CALORIES

PB & FRUIT

makes 1 serving

This PB & Fruit is one smart sandwich. The peanut butter provides filling plant-based protein and healthy fat, and the fresh seasonal fruit adds fiber and antioxidants without the added sugar you typically find in store-bought jams and jellies. Still only three ingredients, this recipe makes the perfect breakfast or lunch . . . or really any-time-of-day munchie.

2 tablespoons natural peanut butter
2 slices reduced-calorie whole-grain bread
   (with no more than 50 calories per slice)
½ cup sliced seasonal fruit, any variety

Spread the peanut butter on 1 slice of bread, add the fruit on top, followed by the second slice of bread, and cut into triangles for easy eating.

---

nutrition information PER SERVING
300 calories ▪ 12 g protein ▪ 17 g total fat (14 g unsaturated, 3 g saturated) ▪ 0 mg cholesterol ▪ 31 g carbs ▪ 6 g fiber 8 g total sugar (8 g natural, 0 g added) ▪ 300 mg sodium

TASTY TWIST Try my Cherry-Chia Jam on page 16 instead of (or in addition to) fresh fruit. It's naturally sweet and loaded with good-for-you ingredients. You can also use any type of nut butter in place of peanut butter. Cashew, almond, soy, and sunflower—they're all delicious and nutritious.

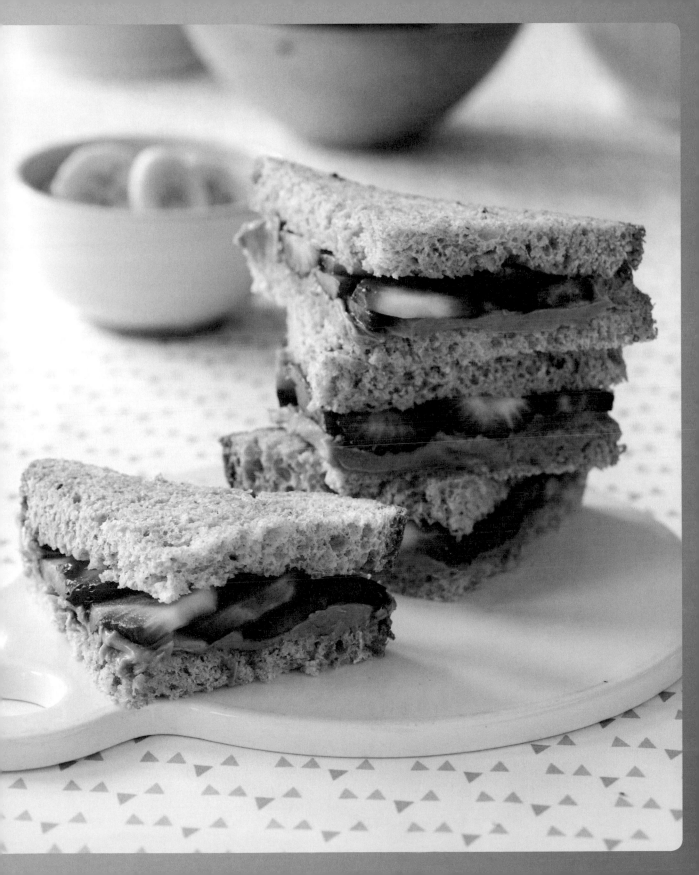

Junk Food

1,290 CALORIES

REUBEN SANDWICH

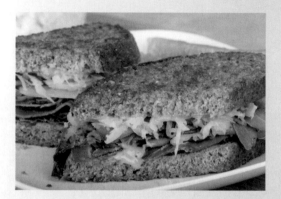

Can you imagine dropping close to 1,300 calories on a sandwich? Order a hearty Reuben sandwich—rye bread, corned beef, Swiss cheese, sauerkraut, and full-fat Russian dressing—from any delicatessen and that's likely what you'll spend.

Instead, try my lightened-up version. It shaves more than 1,000 calories off your typical restaurant version. Cha-ching.

Joy Food

240 CALORIES

TURKEY REUBEN SANDWICH

makes 1 serving

Giving this sandwich a nutritious makeover was a no-brainer. I chose lean turkey over fatty corned beef, piled on plenty of savory sauerkraut, and added enough cheese and Russian dressing to make this sandwich taste like the real deal. While any low-cal, store-bought dressing will work, I encourage you to try my simple DIY Thousand Island recipe (a tasty swap for Russian) on page 120.

> 1 sandwich thin, preferably whole grain
>   (with no more than 100 calories total)
> 2 slices tomato (optional)
> 2 ounces sliced turkey breast (about 4 slices)
> 2 heaping spoonfuls sauerkraut, slightly drained
> 1 ounce reduced-fat Swiss cheese
>   (about 2 thin slices)
> 2 tablespoons Russian dressing (with no more
>   than 50 calories per 2 tablespoons)

Preheat the broiler. Split the sandwich thin and toast it.

Top each half of the toasted sandwich thin with a tomato slice, if desired; turkey; sauerkraut; and 1 slice of Swiss cheese. Place both halves on a baking sheet and place under the broiler until the cheese is melted.

Remove both halves from the oven and top each with 1 tablespoon Russian dressing. Enjoy open-faced.

---

nutrition information PER SERVING
240 calories ▪ 25 g protein ▪ 4.5 g total fat (3.5 g unsaturated, 1 g saturated) ▪ 32 mg cholesterol ▪ 28 g carbs ▪ 3 g fiber 9.5 g total sugar (5 g natural, 4.5 g added) ▪ 900 mg sodium

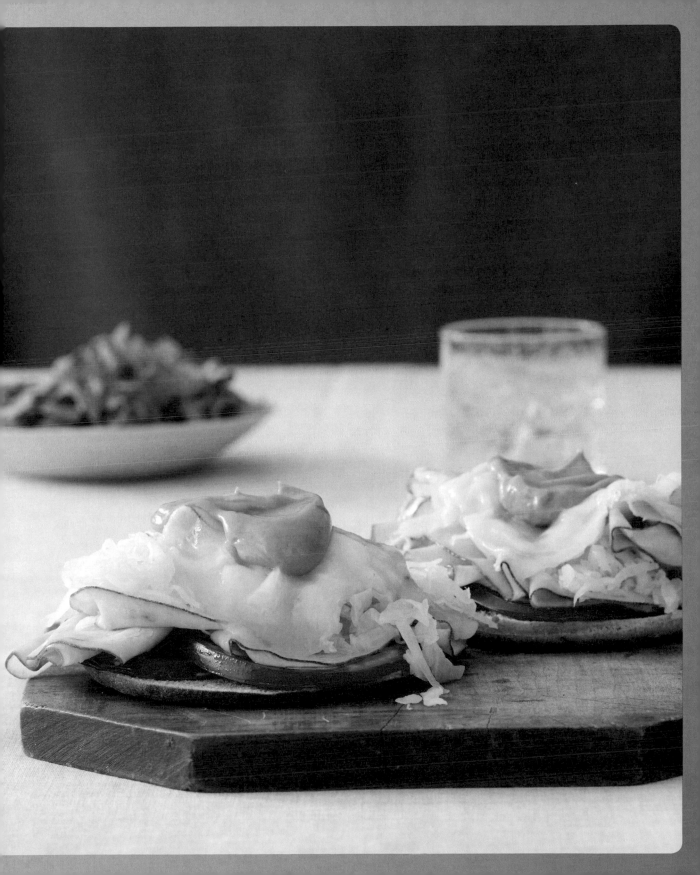

Junk Food

1,570 CALORIES

CHICKEN PARM HERO

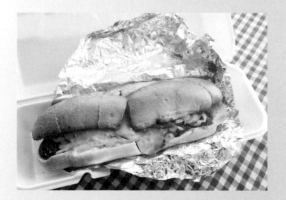

Deep-fried, smothered in cheese, and wrapped in doughy goodness, this Italian classic is pure perfection. Well, that is until you get up from the table feeling stuffed, bloated, and bleh. Reality check: you just consumed more than 1,500 calories and an entire day's worth of salt. Now you're left thinking, *Um, why did I just eat that?*

Get the same flavor without the lousy aftermath by replacing breaded and fried chicken with grilled chicken and scooping out some of the inner dough from your puffy roll. Such simple swaps for significant savings.

Joy Food

320 CALORIES

GRILLED CHICKEN PARM HERO

makes 1 serving

My skinny substitute allows you to indulge in the Italian favorite without suffering a blow to your arteries and waistline. This cheesy creation is downright delicious and a mere 320 calories.

> 1 large whole-grain roll
> 1 thin to medium boneless, skinless chicken breast
> 3 heaping tablespoons marinara sauce, store-bought or homemade
> ¼ cup shredded part-skim mozzarella cheese
> 1 teaspoon grated Parmesan cheese

Preheat the broiler. Line a baking sheet with aluminum foil.

Scoop the insides out of the roll, place the roll on the baking sheet, and lightly toast under the broiler for 1 to 2 minutes. Place the roll on a plate and set aside.

In a pan coated with nonstick oil spray, sauté the chicken until it is no longer pink inside, 3 to 4 minutes per side.

Transfer the chicken to the baking sheet, top with the marinara sauce, mozzarella cheese, and Parmesan cheese. Place under the broiler until the cheese is melted and bubbling. Using a spatula, remove the chicken Parm from the oven and place on a toasted roll.

---

nutrition information PER SERVING
320 calories ▪ 34 g protein ▪ 9 g total fat (5 g unsaturated, 4 g saturated) ▪ 80 mg cholesterol ▪ 22 g carbs ▪ 2 g fiber 3 g total sugar (2 g natural, 1 g added) ▪ 550 mg sodium

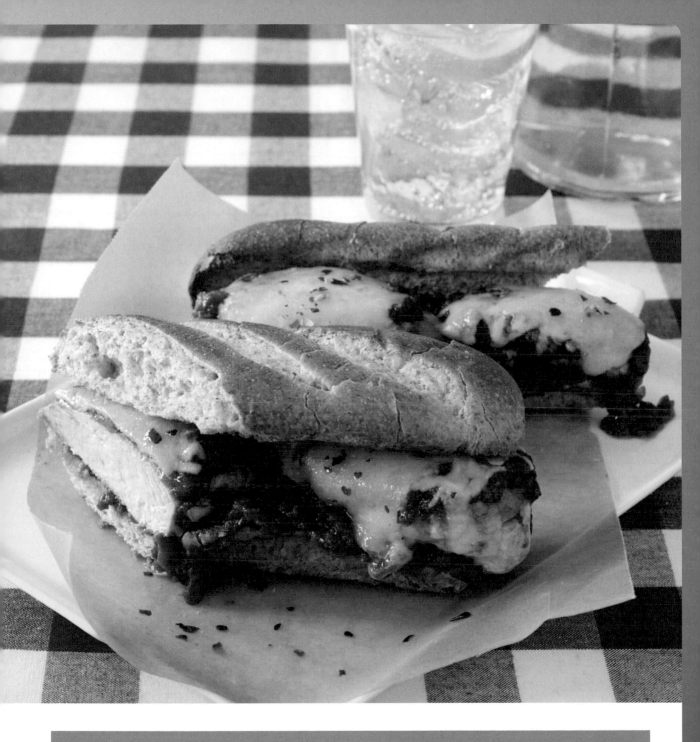

TASTY TWIST For extra flavor, add a dash of oregano and garlic powder on top of the cheese before placing under the broiler. If you like to kick up the heat, like me, you can also add a small pinch of red pepper flakes.

Junk Food

615 CALORIES

LOADED POTATO SOUP

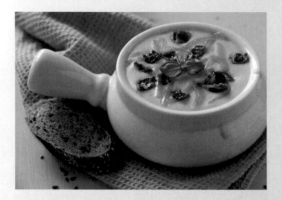

If you've ever enjoyed a bowl of this creamy, spud-filled soup, then you already know that it comes jam-packed with calorific add-ons like bacon, sour cream, and cheddar cheese. Order this at your favorite restaurant, and you could be slurping down more than 600 calories.

My recipe gives you delicious flavor and velvety texture for a fraction of the calories, fat, and carbs.

Joy Food

94 CALORIES

LOADED POTATO SOUP

makes 6 servings

Low in calories and carbs, cauliflower is a vegetable superstar loaded with health-enhancing nutrients. By adding it to this recipe to cut some of the starchy spuds, I've health-ified the ultimate cold-weather comfort food. In fact, I came up with this creation when I was trapped inside on a chilly winter day. It's the perfect cure for cabin fever.

> 1 cup chopped yellow onion (about 1 medium onion)
> 4 cloves garlic, minced, or 1 teaspoon garlic powder
> 3 cups cauliflower florets
> ½ cup shredded carrot
> 1 large potato, cubed (washed well, skin intact)
> 2 cups low-sodium vegetable broth
> 3 tablespoons light or reduced-fat cream cheese
> Salt and pepper to taste

Liberally coat a large pot with nonstick oil spray and warm over medium heat. Add the onion and cook until soft, approximately 5 minutes. Stir frequently to prevent burning. Add more nonstick oil spray if needed.

Add the garlic and cook for 1 to 2 minutes, stirring constantly. Add the cauliflower, carrot, potato, vegetable broth, and 1 cup water. Cover and bring to a boil over high heat.

Reduce the soup to a simmer and cook for 10 minutes with the lid on. Uncover and cook an additional 10 minutes.

Remove the pot from the heat and use an immersion blender to puree the soup until it's smooth. Add the cream cheese and mix vigorously with a spoon until the cream cheese is melted and well blended.

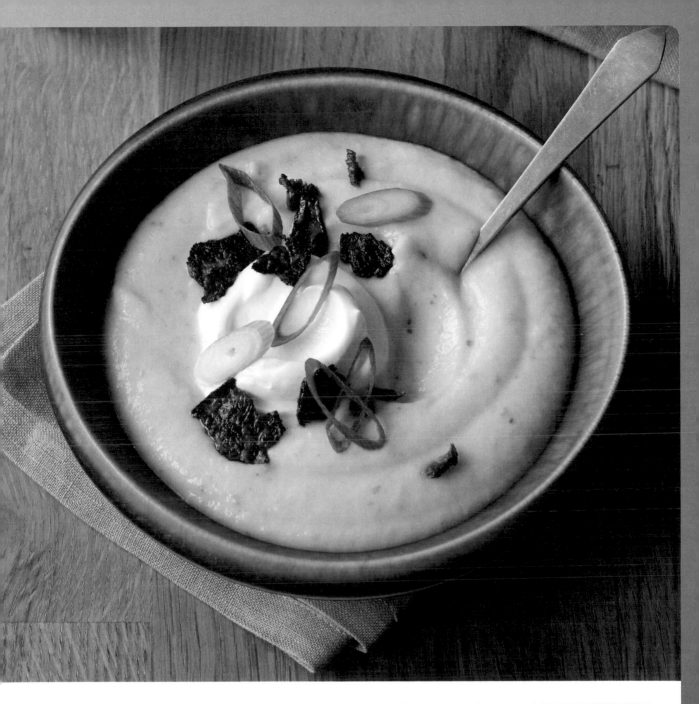

Turn off the heat, season with salt and pepper, and ladle the soup into bowls.

---

nutrition information PER 1-CUP SERVING
94 calories ▪ 3.5 g protein ▪ 1 g total fat (0.25 g unsaturated, 0.75 g saturated) ▪ 0 mg cholesterol ▪ 18 g carbs ▪ 4 g fiber
4 g total sugar (4 g natural, 0 g added) ▪ 110 mg sodium

TASTY TWIST Make this even more flavorful by adding crumbled turkey bacon, nonfat plain Greek yogurt, and sliced scallions.

Junk Food

600 CALORIES

CREAMY TOMATO SOUP

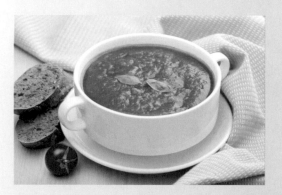

Here's a simple equation to remember: cream = calories, even when the word is followed by a vegetable, as in "Creamy Tomato Soup." While popular canned varieties clock in much lower, a two-cup bowl of the good stuff at a local restaurant can cost around 600 calories, and that's not including the heaps of bread for dipping.

Talk about a *cream* come true (ha . . . I couldn't resist): my slim soup uses a secret ingredient to give you a velvety and smooth texture for just 150 calories per hearty 2-cup serving. Go ahead and have a bowl.

Joy Food

150 CALORIES

CREAMY TOMATO SOUP

makes 4 servings

This dreamy concoction is dairy-free, packed with filling protein, and loaded with antioxidants. By using silken tofu in place of real cream, I managed to significantly slash calories. If you're intimidated by the tofu, take a leap of faith—I swear (scout's honor) that you won't even know it's there.

> 1 tablespoon olive oil
> 1 medium onion, diced
> 2 medium carrots, peeled and chopped
> 2 cloves garlic, crushed
> 3 tablespoons no-salt-added tomato paste
> One 28-ounce can diced fire-roasted tomatoes
> 8 ounces silken tofu, drained and cut into
>   large cubes
> Salt and pepper to taste

Heat the olive oil in a large pot or Dutch oven over medium heat. Add the onion, carrots, and garlic, and sauté until vegetables are tender, about 8 minutes. Add the tomato paste and cook, stirring constantly, for 1 minute.

Add the canned tomatoes. Fill the empty tomato can with water and pour the water into the pot. Bring the soup to a boil, cover the pot, reduce the heat to low, and simmer for 15 minutes. Stir in the tofu and simmer, uncovered, for 15 more minutes.

Puree the soup in small batches in a blender until completely smooth. (Alternatively, use an immersion blender to puree the soup directly in the pot.)

Season with salt and pepper.

---

nutrition information PER 2-CUP SERVING
150 calories ▪ 5.5 g protein ▪ 5 g total fat (4.5 g unsaturated, 0.5 g saturated) ▪ 0 mg cholesterol ▪ 24 g carbs ▪ 5 g fiber 10 g total sugar (10 g natural, 0 g added) ▪ 500 mg sodium

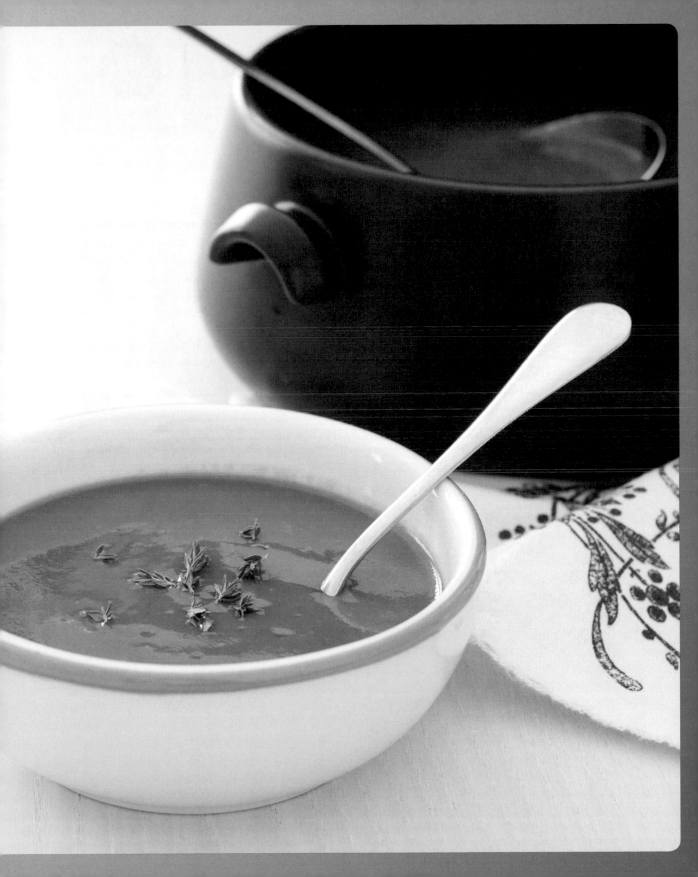

Junk Food

620 CALORIES

FRENCH ONION SOUP

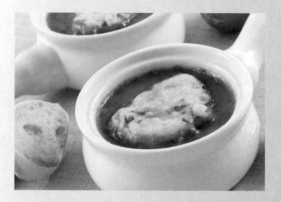

Hearty French onion soup is a classic "warm your heart" appetizer, but it comes at a cost. Order a crock and you'll be spooning down more than 600 calories per serving. It's not necessarily the broth that gets you (although it is typically made with butter), but the caramelized onions, sneaky slices of bread, and the copious amounts of cheese on top.

Instead, slurp skinny with my slimmed-down recipe.

Joy Food

150 CALORIES

FRENCH ONION SOUP

makes 4 servings

There's a lot to love about this cherished soup. Indeed, I'm related to more than a few lifetime members of the French onion soup fan club. Thus, it was my obligation and duty to create a nutritious version that's just as flavorful and full of its signature sweet, caramelized onions and cheese. Grab your spoon and dive in.

> 1 tablespoon olive oil
> 2 large onions, sliced (about 5 cups)
> 2 cloves garlic, minced, or ½ teaspoon garlic powder
> 2 bay leaves
> 2 sprigs fresh thyme
> ¼ teaspoon kosher salt or coarse sea salt
> ½ cup inexpensive red wine (I use cabernet)
> 4 cups low-sodium beef broth
> 4 slices reduced-fat Swiss cheese

Add the olive oil, onions, garlic, bay leaves, thyme, and salt to a large pot. Cook over medium heat until the onions are caramelized to a deep brown color, 25 to 30 minutes. Stir frequently to prevent burning.

Add the red wine and cook until it has evaporated and the onions are dry, about 5 minutes.

Pour in the beef broth, bring the mixture to a boil, reduce the heat to low, and then simmer for 10 minutes.

When ready to eat, turn on the broiler, place four small oven-safe bowls on a baking sheet, ladle the soup into each of the bowls, lay a slice of Swiss cheese over each, and stick the baking sheet in the oven until the cheese is nice and bubbly, 1 to 2 minutes.

nutrition information PER 1-CUP SERVING
150 calories • 12 g protein • 5 g total fat (3.5 g unsaturated, 1.5 g saturated) • 10 mg cholesterol • 10 g carbs • 1.5 g fiber 4 g total sugar (4 g natural, 0 added) • 580 mg sodium

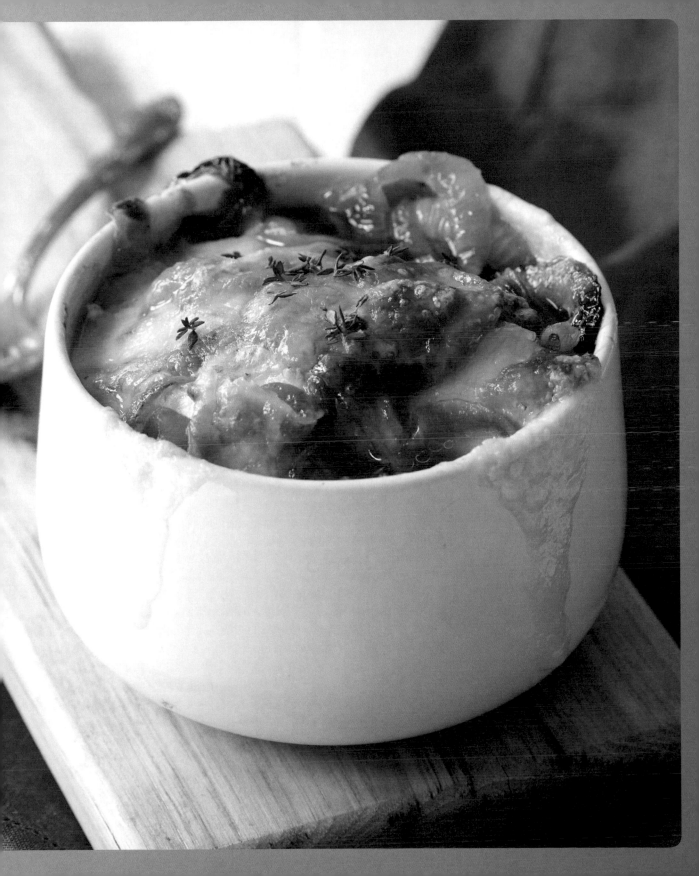

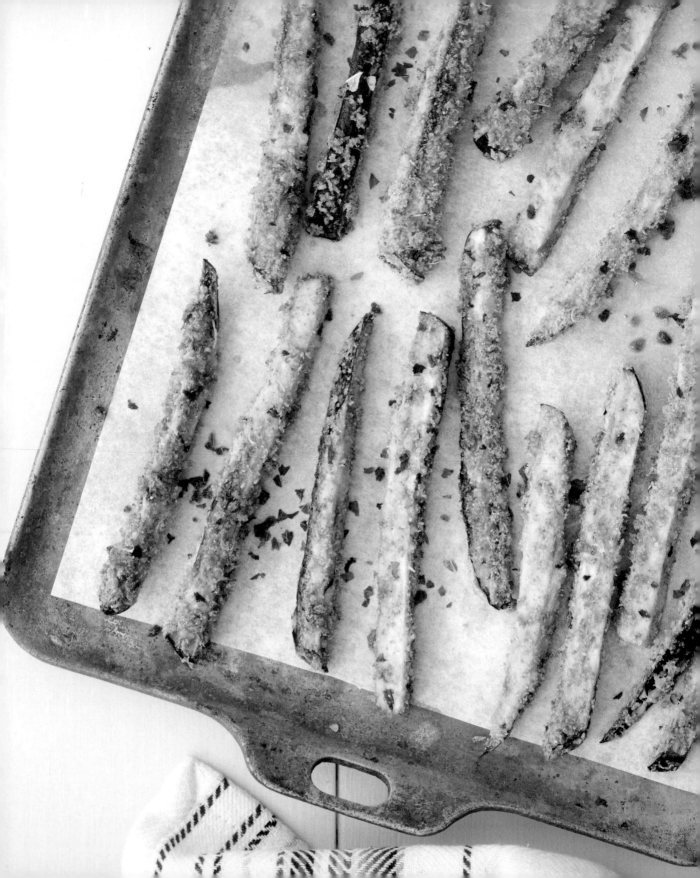

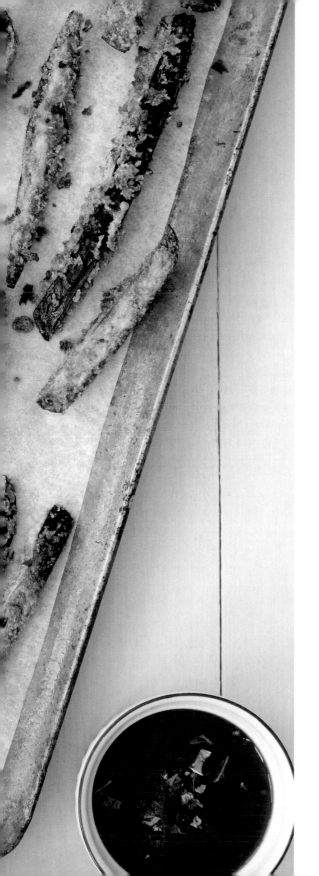

Chapter 4

SLIMMING SIDES, SALADS, AND DRESSINGS

Eat your veggies! You've heard this refrain time and time again, but let's face it, not all veggies are created equal . . . or equally crave-worthy.

For example, a salad could be a dieter's dream or worst nightmare—delicious or bland—depending on what toppings and dressing decorate your greens. Same with your sides; how they're prepared and what ingredients they include could mean your main meal accompaniment is a health-booster or health-buster.

The following recipes marry great taste with great nutrition. Produce can now be proudly positioned to play a starring role on your menu.

Junk Food

BAKED BEANS

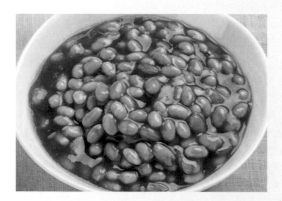

Baked beans are certainly a convenient side (simply pop and pour), but canned versions are often packed with high amounts of sodium and sugar, and potentially a long list of added ingredients.

Not to worry, I managed to re-create this favorite dish, so you can enjoy the benefits of beans without any downsides.

Joy Food

BETTER BAKED BEANS
makes 8 servings

To make my health-ified version, I used just four simple ingredients that you can feel good about feeding your family. As the star of this dish, beans provide a dose of plant-based protein, soluble fiber, and other heart-healthy nutrients. My "secret" ingredient, balsamic vinegar, delivers a serious depth of flavor that takes the dish to another level. This recipe is tangy, sweet, shockingly low in sugar, and a cinch to put together. Go ahead, kick that canned stuff to the curb.

> 1 onion, diced
> Two 15-ounce cans navy, pinto, or cannellini beans, preferably low-sodium, drained and rinsed
> 1 cup barbecue sauce (any brand with no more than 40 calories per 2 tablespoons)
> 1 tablespoon balsamic vinegar

Preheat the oven to 325°F.

Mist a skillet with nonstick oil spray and sauté the onion for 8 to 10 minutes, until soft and translucent. Remove from the heat.

Add the beans, sauce, and vinegar to the onions. Stir until well combined.

Transfer the mixture to a baking dish and bake, uncovered, for 60 minutes, until the sauce is thick.

Serve hot.

---

nutrition information PER ½-CUP SERVING
120 calories ▪ 6 g protein ▪ 0 g total fat (0 g unsaturated, 0 g saturated) ▪ 0 mg cholesterol ▪ 23.5 g carbs ▪ 7 g fiber
5 g total sugar (3 g natural, 2 g added) ▪ 250 mg sodium

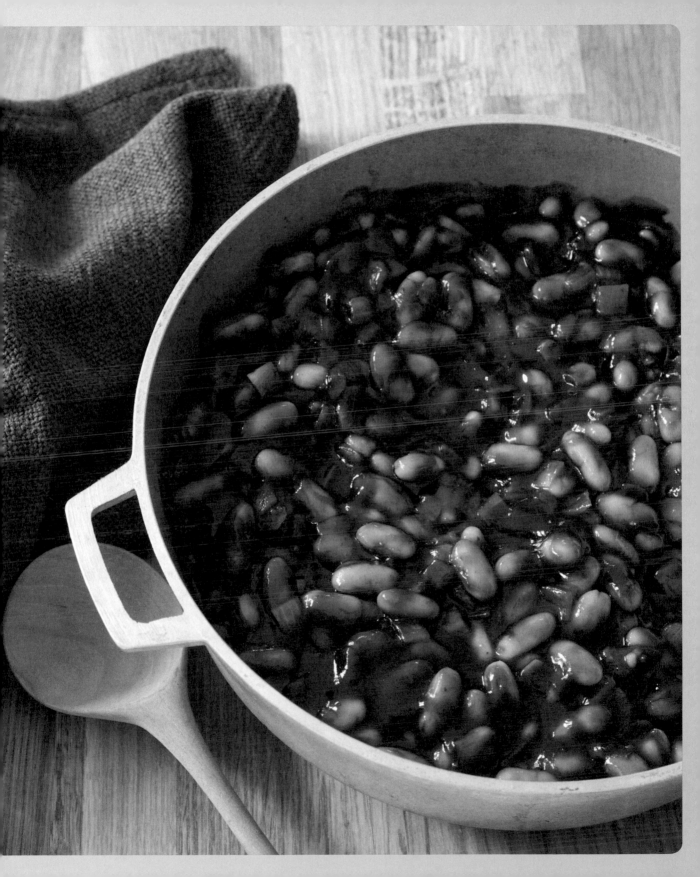

Junk Food

225 CALORIES

MEXICAN CORN ON THE COB

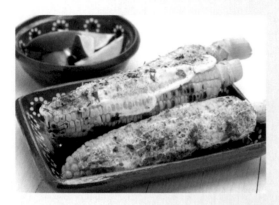

If you've ever tried traditional Mexican corn on the cob (also known as *elote*), then you already know it tastes insanely good. How could it not? It's coated with butter, mayo, and full-fat cheese. Eating one ear of the classic version will set you back 225 calories, no thanks to the fatty fixings. Imagine consuming that much from a side of corn!

But understanding that it's not so easy to give up the spicy, cheesy, slightly charred flavor, I concocted a lower-calorie recipe that I think you'll find just as addictive.

Joy Food

160 CALORIES

MEXICAN CORN ON THE COB

makes 4 servings

Disclaimer: This is no ordinary corn on the cob. In my slimmed-down version, I use light cream cheese and a dash of Parmesan to mimic the rich, creamy texture of the original. I also squeeze on fresh lime for some pizazz and add a pinch of cayenne pepper to kick up the heat. This recipe is the ultimate trifecta: simple to make, low in calories, and a guaranteed party-pleaser. To shuck or not to shuck . . . you decide.

> 4 ears corn
> 4 tablespoons light or reduced-fat cream cheese
> 4 limes
> 4 teaspoons grated Parmesan cheese
> Cayenne pepper to taste

Grill the corn for 15 minutes, rotating every 5 minutes, either in the husk or husks removed and ears wrapped in tinfoil. Alternatively, you can roast the corn in the husks or husks removed and ears wrapped in tinfoil in a 350°F oven by placing them directly on the oven rack for about 30 minutes. The corn is done when it's slightly soft and gives a little beneath the husk or is tender when pierced with a fork.

After the corn is cooked and slightly cooled, peel back each of the husks (if present) and discard or use as a decorative handle for eating. Spread each ear with 1 tablespoon of cream cheese, squeeze on the juice of ½ a lime, and sprinkle on 1 teaspoon of Parmesan cheese and a pinch of cayenne pepper (add more if you like it hot).

Serve with the remaining lime wedges.

---

nutrition information PER SERVING
160 calories ▪ 6 g protein ▪ 4 g total fat (2 g unsaturated, 2 g saturated) ▪ 10 mg cholesterol ▪ 32 g carbs ▪ 4 g fiber 5.5 g total sugar (5.5 g natural, 0 g added) ▪ 110 mg sodium

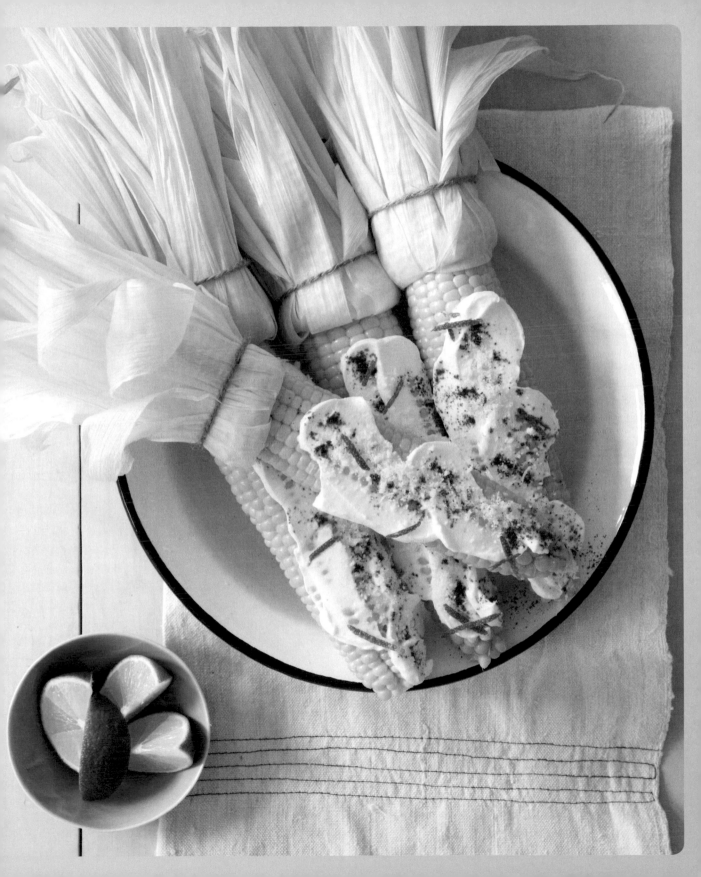

Junk Food

300 CALORIES

MASHED POTATOES

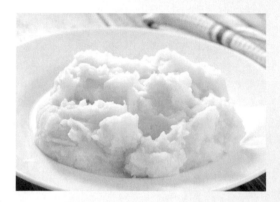

I know what you're thinking: No, please don't touch my mashed potatoes . . . anything but my beloved spuds. They're pure perfection and totally worth the fattening price tag.

Am I close?

But with all that butter, cream (or whole milk), and, of course, the starchy spuds themselves, you're talking about 300 calories and 37 grams of carbs per cup. And that's just for a side dish.

We can do better. My revised recipe delivers big on flavor but comes at a fraction of the calorie-carb cost. Whether you're trying to lose weight or you simply love hot, creamy comfort food, this dish is calling your name.

> **CHOOSE IT TO LOSE IT** Make this mashed potato switch a few times a week and, at the end of the year, you'll trim more than 35,000 calories from your diet—and potentially drop more than 10 pounds.

Joy Food

72 CALORIES

CAULIFLOWER MASHED "POTATOES"

makes 4 servings

Nutrient-dense cauliflower makes the ultimate low-carb substitute for potatoes in this creamy dreamy dish. A cruciferous vegetable, cauliflower has a smooth and velvety texture when pureed, and tastes like a first-class mash when you combine it with broth, cheese, and flavorful seasonings.

1 head cauliflower, cut into florets
¾ cup low-sodium chicken or vegetable broth
1 tablespoon cornstarch
4 ounces (8 tablespoons) fat-free cream cheese
2 tablespoons grated Parmesan or Romano cheese
½ teaspoon garlic powder
¼ teaspoon onion powder
¼ teaspoon paprika
Salt and pepper to taste

Steam the cauliflower over boiling water until fork-tender, about 15 to 20 minutes (or cook in a microwave with 2 tablespoons water for 8 to 10 minutes until very soft). Drain off any liquid. Place the cauliflower in a food processor or blender along with ½ cup broth. Puree on high until smooth. Transfer the puree to a medium saucepan.

In a cup, dissolve the cornstarch in the remaining ¼ cup broth, and add this mixture to the cauliflower puree. Add the cream cheese, Parmesan cheese, garlic powder, onion powder, and paprika. Cook over medium heat, continually stirring, until the puree begins to thicken, 2 to 3 minutes.

Season with salt and pepper. Serve immediately.

---

nutrition information PER 1-CUP SERVING
72 calories ▪ 7.5 g protein ▪ 1 g total fat (0 g unsaturated, 1 g saturated) ▪ 6 mg cholesterol ▪ 8 g carbs ▪ 2 g fiber 3 g total sugar (3 g natural, 0 g added) ▪ 280 mg sodium

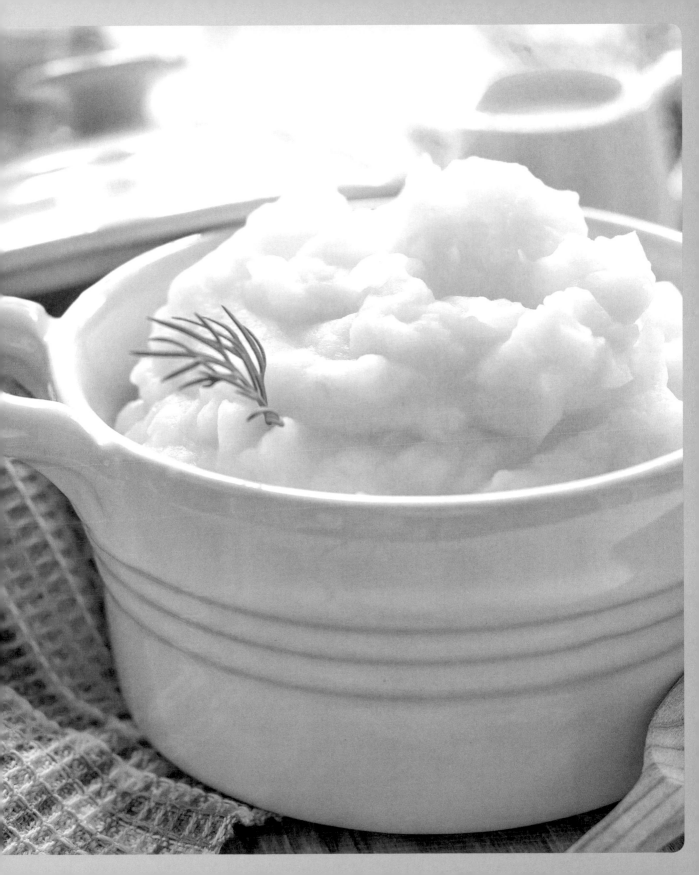

Junk Food

500 CALORIES

LOADED BAKED POTATO

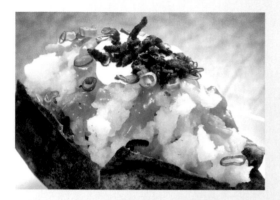

Baked potatoes, sans toppings, can be a healthful food. However, once restaurants stuff 'em full of butter, cheese, sour cream, bacon, and whatever else they can possibly squeeze in, this side dish becomes a nutritional nightmare.

Don't be a stick in the spud. Toss the fatty toppings, and try my slimmer rendition. It's loaded with stuff, all right—nutrients and protein, instead of waist-expanding extras.

Joy Food

226 CALORIES

LOADED BAKED POTATO

makes 1 serving

My recipe redo is a cinch to prepare, and you can easily get creative with add-ons, depending upon what you have in the house. If you're serving a crowd, set up a toppings bar and let everyone build their own special spud. You can lay out all sorts of fixings like chopped tomatoes, diced avocado, corn, cilantro, and crumbled turkey bacon. The assembly is half the fun. For crispy, oven-baked potatoes, follow my instructions below. For quicker cooking, you can always pop them in the microwave. Don't forget to eat the fiber-filled potato skins.

1 medium russet potato
¼ teaspoon kosher salt or coarse sea salt
2 tablespoons cooked black beans
2 tablespoons shredded reduced-fat
   cheddar cheese
2 tablespoons salsa
2 tablespoons nonfat plain Greek yogurt

Preheat the oven to 375°F.

Pierce the potato with a fork about 10 times, mist all sides with nonstick oil spray, and sprinkle on the salt. Place a baking sheet or aluminum foil on a lower rack of the oven to catch drippings. Place the potato directly on the top oven rack and bake for 50 to 60 minutes or until tender.

When the potato is fully baked, split it down the middle and open it slightly. Top it with the beans and cheese and pop it back in the oven or microwave until the cheese is melted. Top with the salsa and Greek yogurt.

---

nutrition information PER SERVING
226 calories • 13 g protein • 3 g total fat (1.5 g unsaturated, 1.5 g saturated) • 10 mg cholesterol • 38 g carbs • 6 g fiber
4 g total sugar (4 g natural, 0 g added) • 640 mg sodium

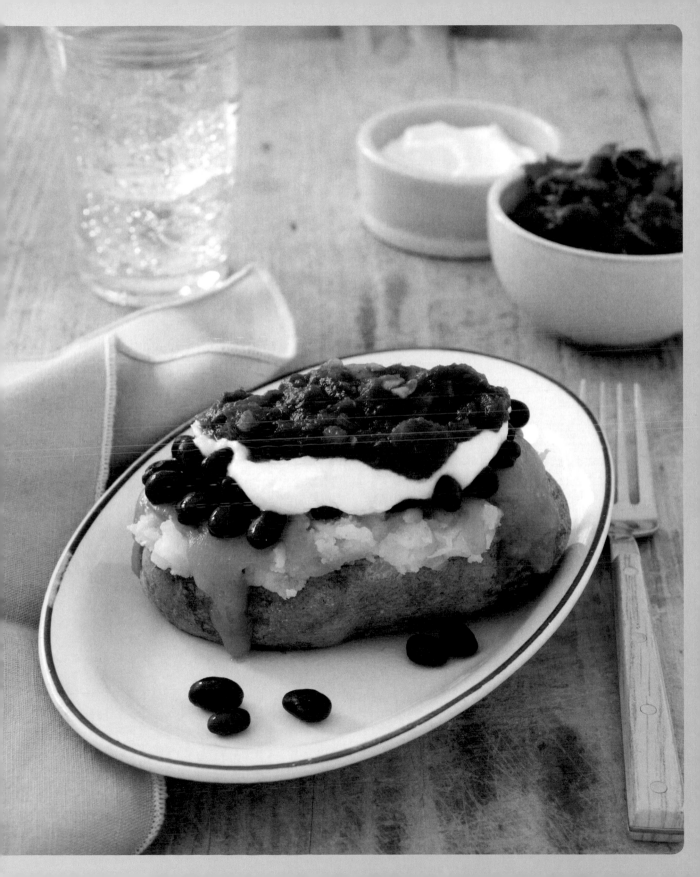

Junk Food

240 CALORIES

CREAMED SPINACH

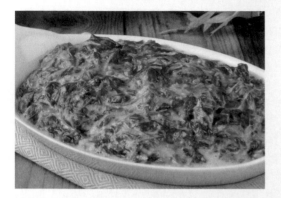

Rich in iron, antioxidants, vitamins, and fiber, spinach is typically a superfood side dish. But beware of the creamed version: one small serving of this velvety veggie can pack as many as 240 calories.

But who can resist? Not me. So I created a skinny rendition that allows you to indulge in this smooth, silky—and yes, creamy!—side anytime you're in the mood.

Joy Food

87 CALORIES

CREAMED SPINACH

makes 4 servings

Here's how to make a steakhouse classic in your own kitchen for a fraction of the calories. Not only is it easy to whip up, but this scrumptious side is packed with good-for-you nutrients, too. Props to Popeye.

> 1 medium shallot, sliced
> 3 cloves garlic, minced
> ¼ teaspoon red pepper flakes
> Two 10-ounce bags fresh spinach, large stems removed, leaves roughly chopped
> 3 ounces (6 tablespoons) light or reduced-fat cream cheese
> ¼ teaspoon kosher salt or coarse sea salt

Coat a large sauté pan with nonstick oil spray. Add the shallot and sauté over medium heat for 5 minutes.

Add the garlic and red pepper flakes and sauté for 1 additional minute.

Add the spinach, a few handfuls at a time, and sauté until wilted, about 3 to 5 minutes.

Add the cream cheese and stir until thoroughly melted and mixed throughout the spinach.

Season the spinach with the salt, and cook 3 to 4 minutes, or until most of the liquid has evaporated.

---

nutrition information PER ¾-CUP SERVING
87 calories ▪ 6 g protein ▪ 4 g total fat (2 g unsaturated, 2 g saturated) ▪ 12 mg cholesterol ▪ 9 g carbs ▪ 3.5 g fiber 2 g total sugar (2 g natural, 0 g added) ▪ 290 mg sodium

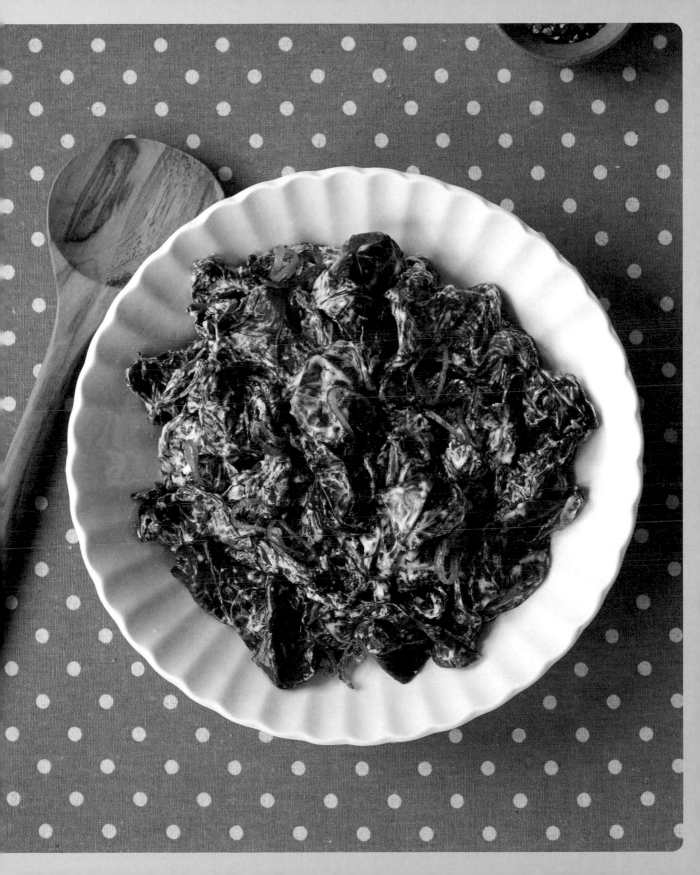

Junk Food

500 CALORIES

FRENCH FRIES

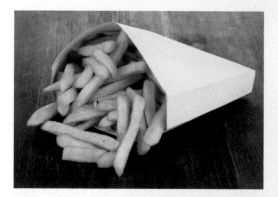

Golden-brown, fried potatoes salted to perfection—drooling yet? The smell alone is irresistible. Unfortunately, the typical large order of fries at your favorite fast-food joint is brimming with 500 calories and heaps of sodium.

But turning this guilty pleasure into a healthier side is easier than you may think: the secret is skipping the fryer (you will not miss it—I swear!) and using nutrient-packed sweet potatoes (although you can certainly use white potatoes if the sweet ones aren't your thing).

> **CHOOSE IT TO LOSE IT** Make this French fry trade three times a week and, by the end of the year, you'll save 62,000 calories—and potentially shed 18 pounds.

Joy Food

100 CALORIES

SWEET POTATO FRIES

makes 4 servings

Crispy and crunchy, my oven-baked fries are every bit as delicious as the deep-fried kind. By using sweet potatoes as the base, these fries offer something the average French fry doesn't—plenty of beta-carotene, an antioxidant that keeps your eyes, skin, and hair vibrant and healthy.

2 sweet potatoes (about 8 ounces each)
1 teaspoon cumin
¼ teaspoon cayenne pepper (skip if you're not a fan of heat)
1¼ teaspoons kosher salt or coarse sea salt
¼ teaspoon cinnamon
Ground black pepper to taste

Preheat the oven to 400°F. Coat a large baking sheet with nonstick oil spray and set aside.

Slice off the ends of the potatoes and cut the potatoes in half lengthwise. Cut each half into wedges or strips (approximately ¼ inch thick). Spread the fries out in a single layer on the baking sheet and spray liberally with nonstick oil spray. Sprinkle the fries evenly with seasonings.

Bake the fries for 20 minutes, flipping them halfway through. To finish, set the oven to broil and cook for 5 or more minutes (depending on how brown and crispy you like your fries—watch closely so they don't burn).

---

nutrition information PER SERVING
100 calories ▪ 2 g protein ▪ 0 g total fat (0 g unsaturated, 0 g saturated) ▪ 0 mg cholesterol ▪ 23 g carbs ▪ 3.5 g fiber
4.5 g total sugar (4.5 g natural, 0 g added sugar)
410 mg sodium

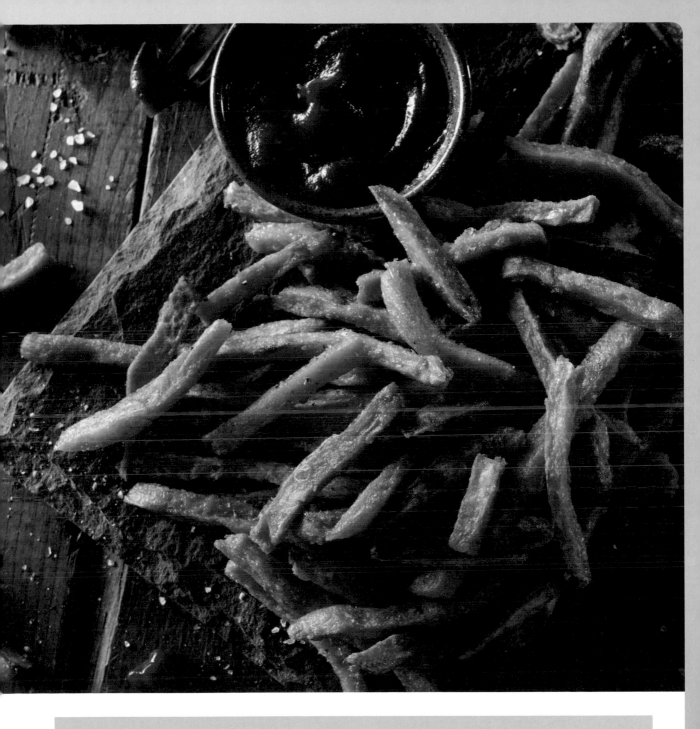

TASTY TWIST Sweet potatoes aren't your only healthy option. Jicama (pronounced hick-ama) is a crunchy, sweet, nutty root vegetable. You can make jicama fries by simply slicing jicama into "fry-like" strips, adding a squeeze of lime juice, and seasoning with salt and pepper. For a fiery twist, add a dash of chili powder. The end result is a delicious and refreshing no-bake treat for only 45 calories per 1-cup serving.

Junk Food 885 CALORIES

FRIED ZUCCHINI

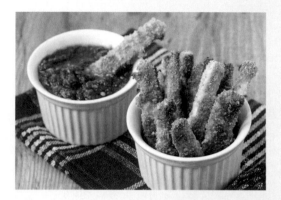

We've all heard that a veggie appetizer can help cut calories when eating out. Generally this means virtuous green vegetables that aren't dipped in eggs, battered in refined starch, and then deep-fried in a vat of oil, soaking up more than you even want to know about (trust me, you don't want to know). Therefore, an order of fried zucchini sticks—weighing in at more than 800 calories—wouldn't make the cut.

My Eggplant Fries give you the same finger-food experience for markedly fewer calories. What's more, they've scored lots of flattering comments like "absolutely amazing!" and "OMG, these are addictive!" from people who have made the recipe. Dunk them in warm marinara sauce and your taste buds will be dancing with appreciation.

Joy Food 220 CALORIES

EGGPLANT FRIES

makes 4 servings

I tested this recipe makeover for the first time live on the *Today* show (pretty brave, huh?). It was the ultimate challenge from my good pal Kathie Lee Gifford—and I'm relieved to report that she flipped for them. In fact, she wouldn't move on to the next recipe demo and instead remained glued to my eggplant plate, munching away. Best. Segment. Ever.

Serve them up as a snack for your family or as an appetizer for company—either way, they will get gobbled up in no time.

    1 medium eggplant
    ½ cup whole-grain flour
    3 egg whites
    1 cup panko bread crumbs, preferably whole-grain
    1 cup grated Parmesan cheese
    1 tablespoon olive oil
    1¼ teaspoons kosher salt or coarse sea salt
    ½ teaspoon ground black pepper
    1 teaspoon garlic powder
    1 teaspoon dried basil
    Marinara sauce, store-bought or
       homemade (optional)

Preheat the oven to 450°F.

Line two baking sheets with aluminum foil and lightly spray each with nonstick oil spray. Set aside.

Cut off both ends of the eggplant, and then cut the eggplant in half crosswise. Slice the eggplant lengthwise into sticks ½ inch thick and 3 inches long.

Place the flour onto a dish. In a separate shallow bowl, whisk the egg whites until combined (this is important in order to get an even coating). In a separate bowl, combine the bread crumbs, Parmesan cheese, olive oil, salt, pepper, garlic powder, and basil.

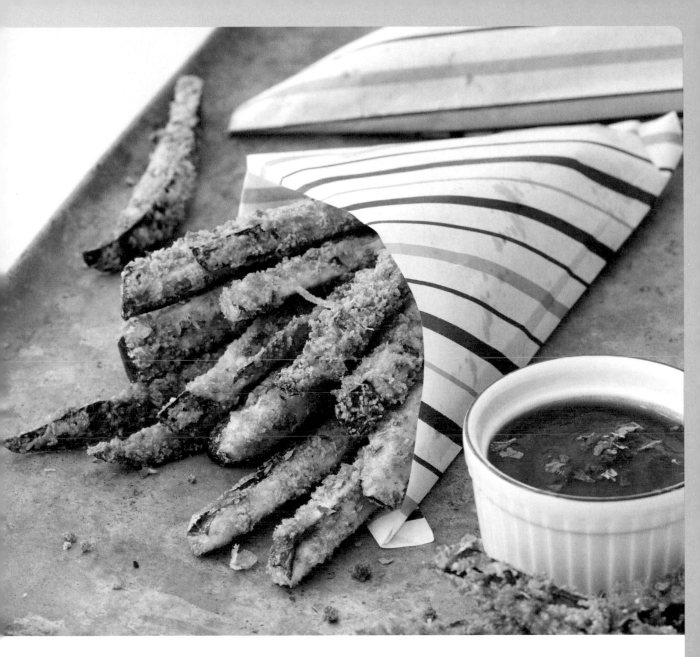

Dredge the eggplant slices lightly in the flour and tap gently to remove the excess. Then, working in batches, dunk the floured eggplant fries into the egg to coat, and then toss in the bread crumb–Parmesan mixture, pressing gently to make sure it adheres.

Place the fries on the prepared baking sheets, leaving space between the fries. Bake for 15 minutes, turn the fries over, rotate the baking sheets, and bake for an additional 5 minutes, or until golden brown on all sides.

Serve with warm marinara sauce for dunking, if desired.

Note: Fries bake best on the top level of the oven. For a crispier texture, make sure all the fries get a turn on the top rack closest to the broiler.

nutrition information PER SERVING
220 calories ▪ 14 g protein ▪ 7.5 g total fat (4 g unsaturated, 3.5 g saturated) ▪ 40 mg cholesterol ▪ 27 g carbs ▪ 7 g fiber
4 g total sugar (4 g natural, 0 g added) ▪ 800 mg sodium

Junk Food

150 CALORIES

GARLIC BREAD

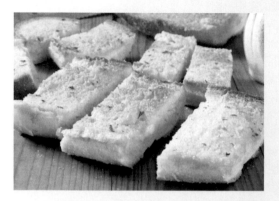

Garlicky, buttery, and oh so good, there's no denying the appeal of toasty garlic bread. It's finger-lickin' divine. But at 150 calories a slice, it will dent your diet and assault your arteries—especially because nobody stops at one piece.

I simplified it—and slimmed it down—by focusing on the heroic and healthy headliner: garlic. And boy, is it ever delish.

Joy Food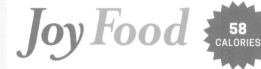

58 CALORIES

GARLIC BREAD

makes 4 servings

When you think about it, garlic bread really is all about the garlic. So I nixed the unnecessary extras (aka butter, white bread, cheese) and played up the breathtaking bulb. When you roast garlic to perfection, it transforms to a soft, spreadable, mouthwatering consistency.

And pass on the white bread; go for a whole-grain baguette for a shot of fiber and phytonutrients, as I've done in the recipe below. Finally, consider serving with a mint.

> 1 head garlic
> 1 teaspoon olive oil
> Salt and pepper to taste
> 4 whole-grain baguette slices

Preheat the oven to 400°F.

Trim the top off the head of garlic to expose the tops of the cloves, drizzle oil over them, sprinkle them with salt and pepper, and wrap the whole thing in aluminum foil. Roast the garlic in the oven for about 30 minutes, until the garlic is soft.

Toast the baguette slices.

Remove the garlic from the oven and gently squeeze the cloves from the skin. They should be very soft. Spread about 3 cloves on each slice of toasted baguette.

---

nutrition information PER SERVING
58 calories ▪ 2 g protein ▪ 1.5 g total fat (1.5 g unsaturated, 0 g saturated) ▪ 0 mg cholesterol ▪ 9 g carbs ▪ 1 g fiber 0 g total sugar (0 g natural, 0 g added) ▪ 74 mg sodium

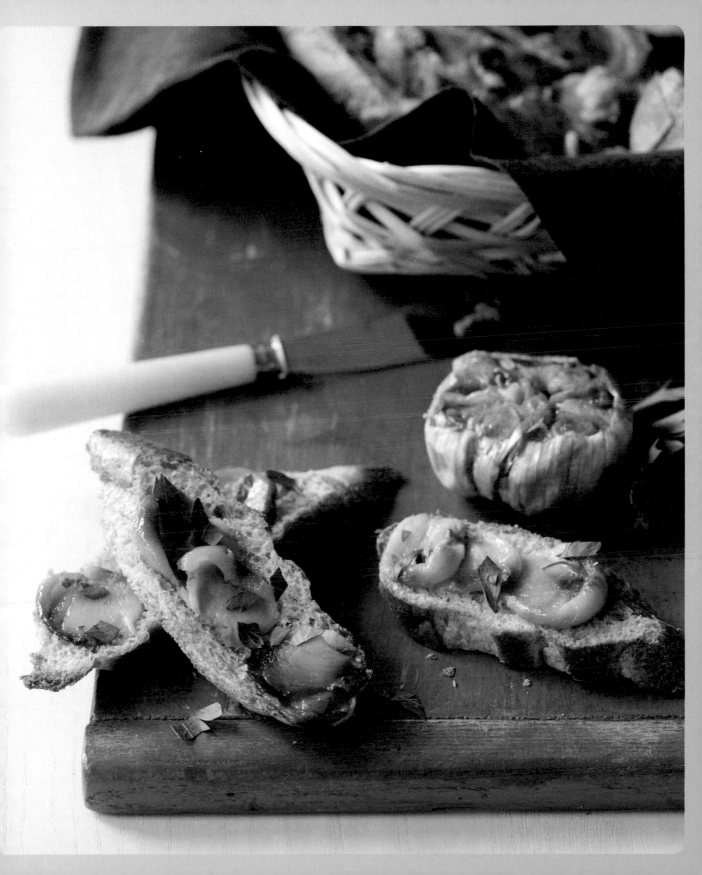

Junk Food

350 CALORIES

POTATO SALAD

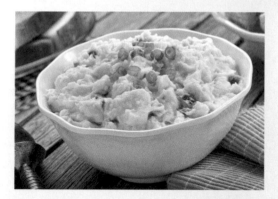

Don't be fooled by the name—this "salad" is very different from a bowl filled with leafy greens. The usual starchy potato salad at your family barbecue is undoubtedly drenched with fattening mayo. Just a few heaping spoonfuls—about 1 cup—of the spud-filled side can set you back 350 calories.

My twist on this classic recipe has all the potato-y goodness without the unnecessary gunk. And by adding Greek yogurt to the mix, my lightened-up version provides an extra dose of protein that will help keep you feeling full and satisfied, which means more self-control by the time dessert rolls around. Double score.

Joy Food

50 CALORIES

POTATO SALAD BITES

makes 13 servings

Whip up a batch of these perfectly portioned super-spuds for your next cookout or picnic. Top them with my lemony-dill yogurt for a ridiculously tasty dish that will be sure to please your potato-loving friends. Bonus: no eating utensils required.

13 small red potatoes (24-ounce bag)
½ teaspoon kosher salt or coarse sea salt
Ground black pepper to taste
½ cup nonfat plain Greek yogurt
1 tablespoon fresh lemon juice
½ teaspoon dried dill or chopped fresh dill

Preheat the oven to 450°F.

Wash the potatoes well, and then slice them in half lengthwise, leaving the skin on. For larger potatoes, cut them so they are similar in size to the others; this will allow them to cook evenly.

Place the potatoes in a baking dish, mist them with nonstick oil spray, and season them with salt and pepper. Toss well and arrange potatoes in a single layer (cut side up). Bake for 25 minutes or until a fork easily pierces the larger potato pieces.

Allow the potatoes to cool for at least 40 minutes. Or store in the fridge to keep chilled for when you're ready to serve.

In the meantime, make the lemon-dill yogurt topping by mixing the Greek yogurt, lemon juice, and dill in a small bowl.

Right before serving, top each potato half (chilled or room temperature) with a dollop of the lemon-dill yogurt dressing.

---

nutrition information PER SERVING OF 2 POTATO HALVES WITH TOPPING ▪ 50 calories ▪ 2 g protein ▪ 0 g total fat (0 g unsaturated, 0 g saturated) ▪ 0 mg cholesterol ▪ 10 g carbs 2 g fiber ▪ 1 g total sugar (1 g natural, 0 g added) ▪ 55 mg sodium

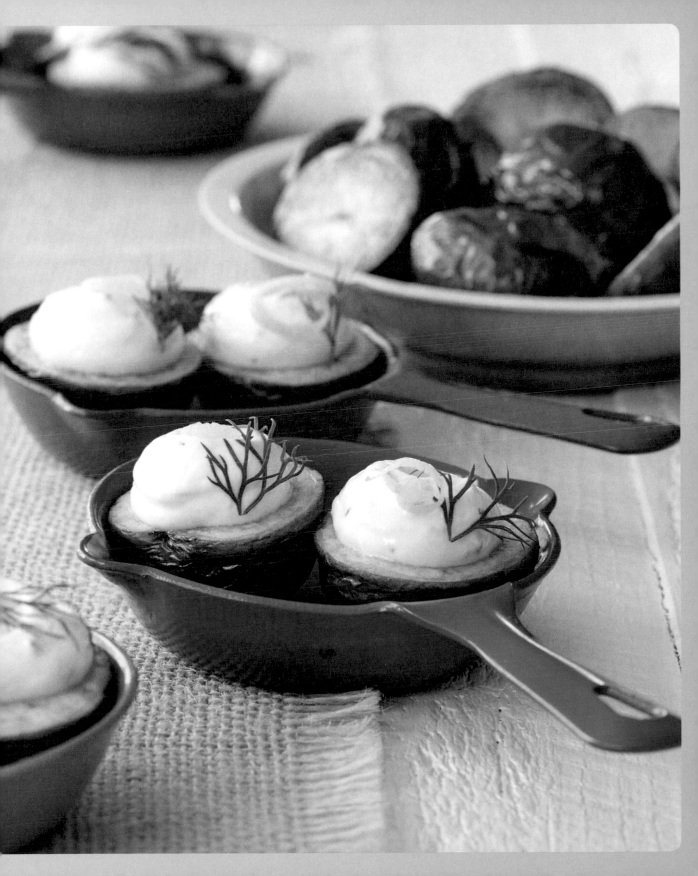

Junk Food

290 CALORIES

COLESLAW

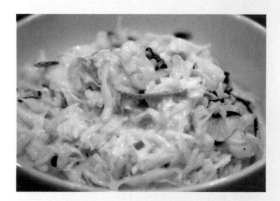

What's a barbecue without crunchy coleslaw? By far, it's one of my favorite sides at cookouts. But here's the catch: Traditional versions of this delicious dish douse innocent shredded cabbage in heaps of fatty mayo. The end result is a mayonnaise soup (often with added sugar) that packs 290 calories per cup.

Instead, mix up my creamy version and skip the store-bought slaw. I promise, you—or your guests—won't miss the heavy original.

Joy Food

50 CALORIES

COLESLAW

makes 6 servings

My better-for-you recipe uses scallions and dried cranberries for fantastic flavor, a pop of color, and a dose of nutrition. By using smaller amounts of low-fat mayo, this simple slaw lets the powerful taste of carrots and cabbage (a cruciferous superstar that may reduce the risk of certain cancers) shine through. Dig in and reap the benefits.

> 4 cups shredded cabbage (see note)
> 2 cups shredded carrots (see note)
> ½ cup chopped scallions (green onions)
> ¼ cup dried cranberries
> ¼ cup low-fat mayonnaise
> 1 tablespoon apple cider vinegar or orange juice
> 1 teaspoon Dijon mustard
> ½ teaspoon kosher salt or coarse sea salt
> Ground black pepper to taste

Combine all the ingredients in a large bowl and toss to mix.

Note: You may use 6 cups store-bought preshredded vegetable blend in place of the cabbage and carrots.

---

nutrition information PER 1-CUP SERVING
50 calories ▪ 1 g protein ▪ 1 g total fat (1 g unsaturated, 0 g saturated) ▪ 0 mg cholesterol ▪ 10 g carbs ▪ 3 g fiber
7 g total sugar (4 g natural, 3 g added) ▪ 236 mg sodium

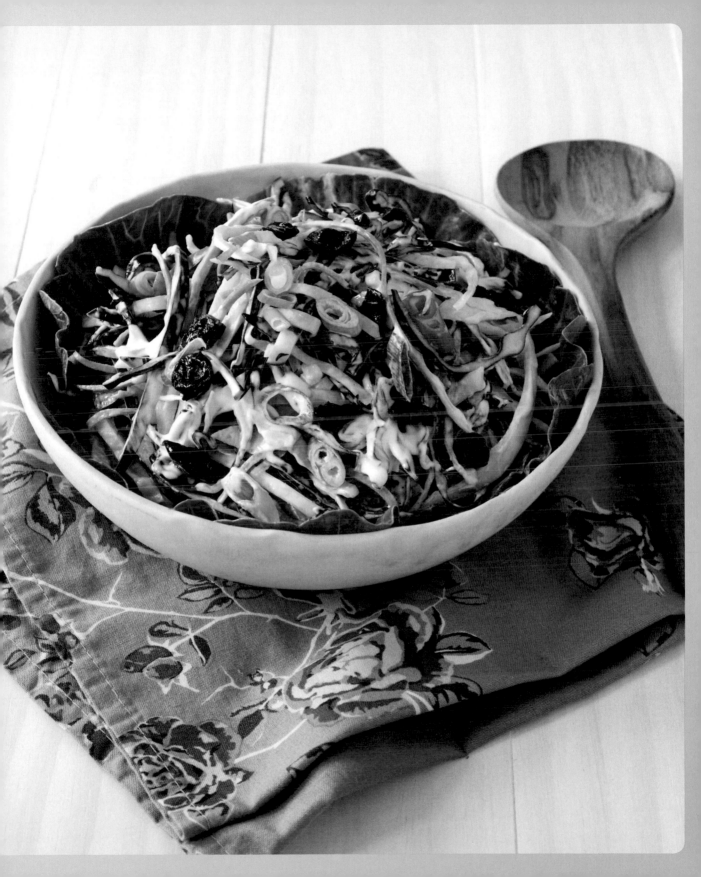

Junk Food

980 CALORIES

CHICKEN CAESAR SALAD

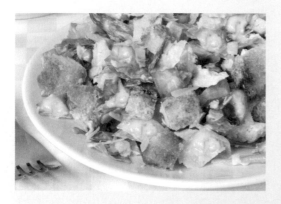

You order a chicken Caesar salad at a restaurant thinking you're making a lighter pick, when in reality, you'd have been better off with a burger. No joke! A typical Caesar salad with grilled chicken, croutons, Parmesan cheese, and creamy dressing will set you back nearly 1,000 calories, whereas an old-fashioned hamburger on a bun would cost you about 550.

If you're craving Caesar, go ahead and order one, but request the dressing on the side (it's by far the biggest offender), and then be stingy and use only about 2 tablespoons' worth. Another option: make your own salad at home using my simple recipe.

Joy Food

350 CALORIES

CHICKEN CAESAR SALAD

makes 1 serving

Enjoy the delicious classic flavors of Caesar salad—Parmesan shavings and all—without blowing a day's worth of calories in one sitting with this slim-style rendition.

> 2 cups chopped romaine lettuce
> 4 ounces cooked (unbreaded) chicken, cut into strips
> 2 tablespoons reduced-calorie Caesar dressing (store-bought or my Caesar Dressing on page 122)
> 1 ounce shaved or grated Parmesan cheese
> Ground black pepper to taste

Top the lettuce with the chicken and dressing, and toss to coat. Sprinkle on the cheese and season with pepper.

nutrition information PER SERVING
350 calories ▪ 47 g protein ▪ 11 g total fat (5 g unsaturated, 6 g saturated) ▪ 140 mg cholesterol ▪ 14 g carbs ▪ 2 g fiber 5 g total sugar (4 g natural, 1 g added) ▪ 960 mg sodium

> **TASTY TWIST** Missing the croutons? Toss in a handful of roasted chickpeas or toasted, chopped walnuts for a lower-carb and higher-fiber crunch; ¼ cup chickpeas adds 60 calories, 3 grams protein, and 3.5 grams fiber. 2 tablespoons walnuts adds 95 calories, 2 grams protein, and 1 gram fiber.

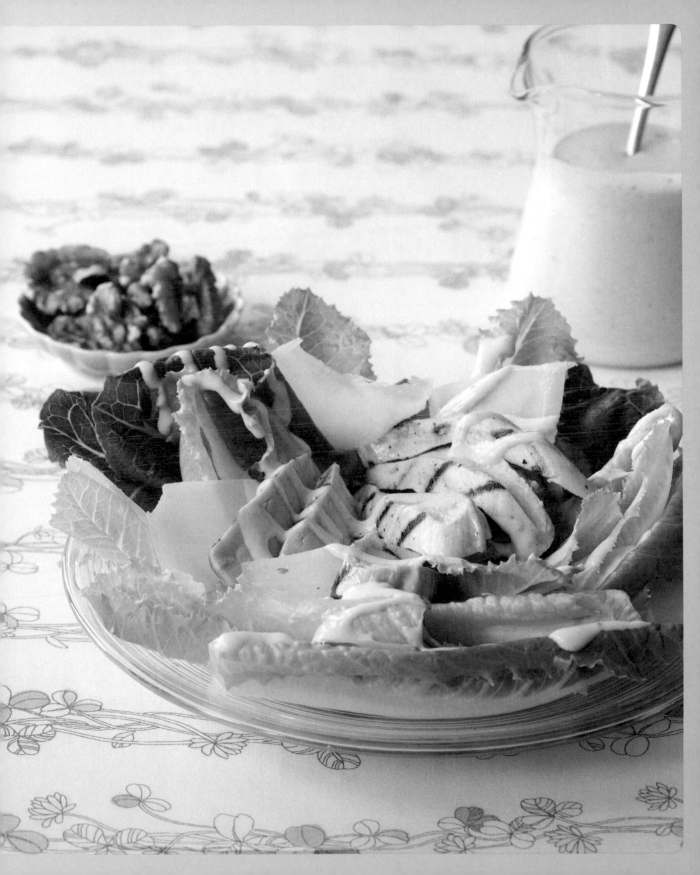

Junk Food

150 CALORIES

RANCH DRESSING

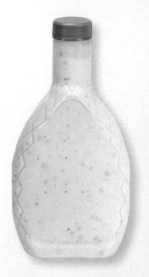

It's no surprise that ranch tops the list as the nation's most popular salad dressing. Rich, velvety, and full of flavor, it's like bottled magic. I've seen the most veggie-averse kids devour broccoli, carrots, and cauliflower simply because the produce picks were covered with the good stuff. Unfortunately, it comes at a cost: 150 calories per 2 tablespoons.

Not mine! For just 22 calories, you (and your little ones) can enjoy it totally guilt-free.

Joy Food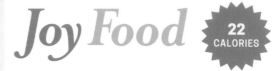

22 CALORIES

RANCH DRESSING

makes 8 servings

Finally, a rich and flavorful ranch dressing you can pour with total abandon. This zesty rendition is super thick, so it works as both a salad topper and a yummy dip for veggies. For a thinner, pourable dressing, just add a bit more buttermilk.

  ½ cup fat-free sour cream
  2 tablespoons low-fat mayonnaise
  2 tablespoons low-fat buttermilk
  1 tablespoon fresh lemon juice
  ¼ teaspoon ground black pepper
  ¾ teaspoon onion powder
  ¼ teaspoon garlic powder
  1 scallion (green onion), finely chopped
  1 tablespoon finely chopped fresh parsley

Combine all the ingredients in a bowl and stir well to combine.

---

nutrition information PER 2-TABLESPOON SERVING
22 calories • 1 g protein • 0.5 g total fat (0.5 g unsaturated, 0 g saturated) • 0 mg cholesterol • 4 g carbs • 0 g fiber
1.5 g total sugar (1.5 g natural, 0 g added) • 50 mg sodium

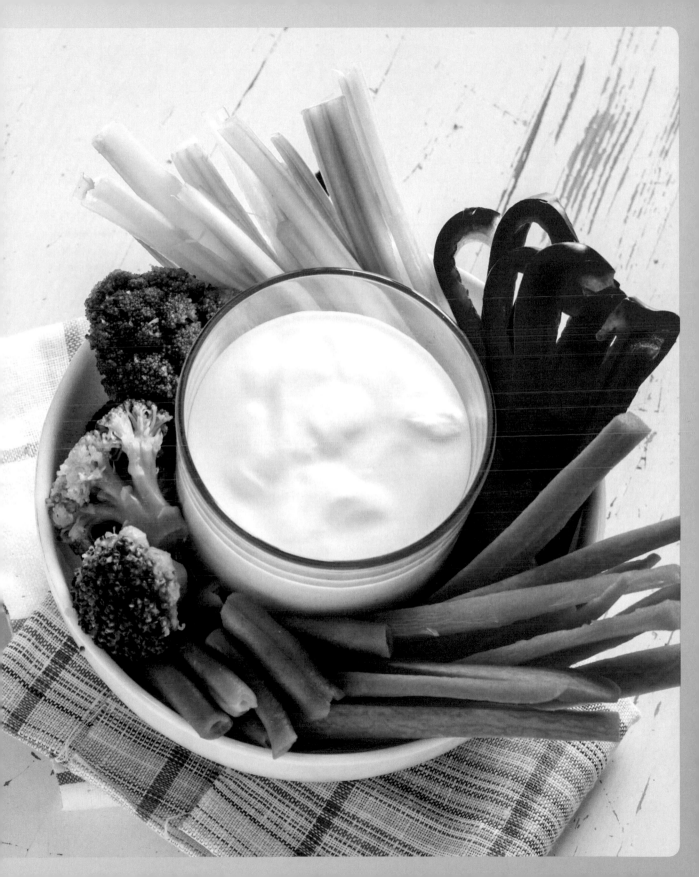

Junk Food

BALSAMIC VINAIGRETTE

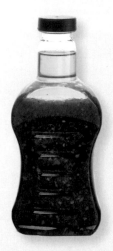

Store-bought salad dressings are typically loaded with calories and sodium. Balsamic vinaigrette, contrary to its healthy reputation, is no different. It can contain up to 145 calories and more than 300 milligrams of sodium in a measly 2-tablespoon serving. Pour that (or more) over a bowl of innocent leafy greens, and you'll lose the low-cal, nutrient-packed advantage.

Luckily, it's easy to make your own tasty dressing with ingredients you probably already have in your kitchen. The health payoff is definitely worth a bit of extra effort, and you can truly enjoy a delectable, light lunch.

Joy Food

BALSAMIC VINAIGRETTE

makes 8 servings

No need to drown your greens in heavy, fattening dressings. If you're a balsamic vinaigrette fan like me, I encourage you to try my simple DIY recipe. Mix together just a few everyday ingredients—with balsamic vinegar playing a starring role, of course—and then get ready to say hello to your new go-to salad topper.

- ½ cup balsamic vinegar (choose a good-quality, aged vinegar if possible)
- 3 tablespoons extra-virgin olive oil
- 1 tablespoon Dijon mustard
- 1 teaspoon honey
- 1 teaspoon garlic powder

Combine all the ingredients plus ¼ cup water in a jar or container with a screw-on lid. Screw on the lid and shake the container vigorously until everything is well combined.

Note: You can store this dressing in the refrigerator in the same container you prepped it in. Just shake the container vigorously before each use to mix the ingredients.

---

nutrition information PER 2-TABLESPOON SERVING
55 calories ▪ 0 g protein ▪ 5 g total fat (4.5 g unsaturated, 0.5 g saturated) ▪ 0 mg cholesterol ▪ 3 g carbs ▪ 0 g fiber 1 g total sugar (0 g natural, 1 g added) ▪ 40 mg sodium

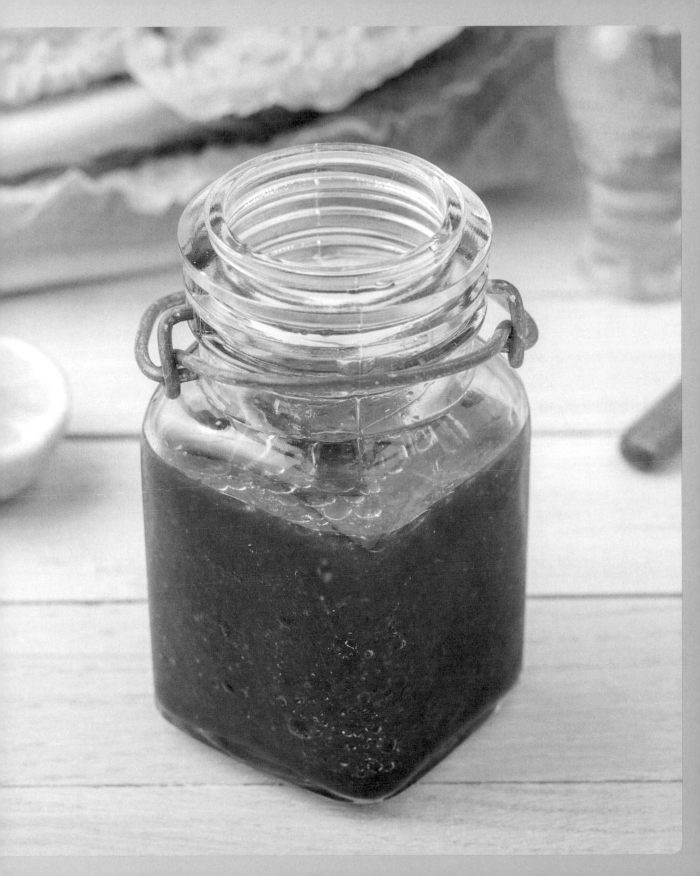

*Junk*Food 110 CALORIES

GREEN GODDESS DRESSING

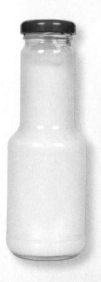

Looking to top off your greens with something green? Beware of the green goddess. The thick salad topper consists of herbs (hence the green hue) mixed with mayo, sour cream, and anchovy paste. There are as many as 110 calories per 2 tablespoons—and most of us use 4 to 6. Bet you're doing the math in your head . . . scary.

Use my light version instead for a flavorful salad that tastes truly heavenly.

*Joy*Food 25 CALORIES

GREEN GODDESS DRESSING

makes 12 servings

Other dressings will be green with envy because this salad topper offers a delicious taste for a negligible number of calories. It doubles as a dip for crudités, too. Gotta love multitasking munchies.

- ½ cup mashed ripe avocado (about ¾ of a medium avocado)
- 3 scallions (green onions), roughly chopped (about ½ cup)
- ½ cup roughly chopped fresh basil
- 2 tablespoons fresh lemon juice
- 1 clove garlic, minced, or ¼ teaspoon garlic powder
- 1 teaspoon kosher salt or coarse sea salt
- ½ teaspoon ground black pepper
- ½ cup light sour cream
- 1 teaspoon anchovy paste (optional)

Place all the ingredients plus 2 tablespoons water in a food processor or powerful blender, and puree until everything is thoroughly combined and smooth.

---

nutrition information PER 2-TABLESPOON SERVING
25 calories ▪ 1 g protein ▪ 1.5 g total fat (1.5 g unsaturated, 0 g saturated) ▪ 0 mg cholesterol ▪ 2.5 g carbs ▪ 1 g fiber 1 g total sugar (1 g natural, 0 g added) ▪ 105 mg sodium

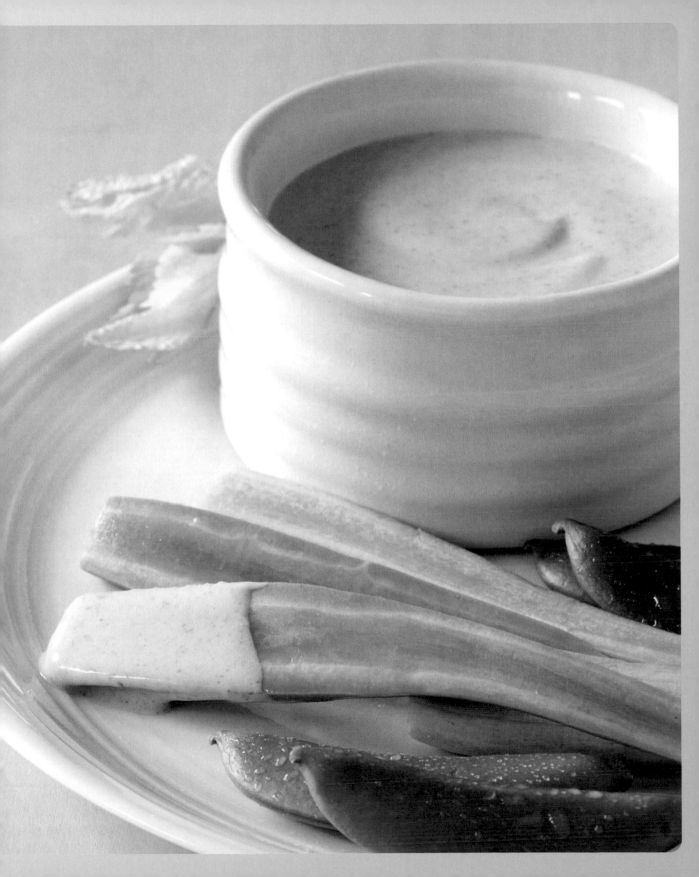

Junk Food

FRENCH DRESSING

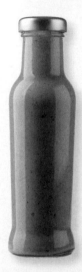

French dressing is a go-to for salad lovers, but like so many other store-bought bottles, it can tip the scales. Consider that 2 tablespoons will add 130 calories to an otherwise light lunch . . . pour on double or triple that amount, and your diet-friendly salad becomes a belly-bloating bowl.

You'll never be overdressed with my 20-calorie rendition. By simply replacing the traditional oil used with creamy yogurt and incorporating classic ingredients like paprika and vinegar, you can now enjoy a fit and flavorful feast.

Joy Food

FRENCH DRESSING

makes 8 servings

Drizzle on my new and improved French Dressing to add delicious flavor without dousing your bowl with lots of extra fat and calories. This recipe couldn't be any easier. Mix up ketchup, yogurt, vinegar, and paprika, along with a few mainstay seasonings, and you have a light dressing that's every bit as satisfying as the real McCoy.

- ¼ cup ketchup
- ½ cup nonfat plain Greek yogurt
- 1 teaspoon honey
- 1 teaspoon Worcestershire sauce
- 2 tablespoons rice wine vinegar
- 1 teaspoon paprika
- ¼ teaspoon onion powder
- 1 teaspoon kosher salt or coarse sea salt
- ¼ teaspoon ground black pepper

Combine all the ingredients plus 1 tablespoon water in a small bowl and stir to combine.

---

nutrition information PER 2-TABLESPOON SERVING
20 calories • 2 g protein • 0 g total fat (0 g unsaturated, 0 g saturated) • 0 mg cholesterol • 3.5 g carbs • 0 g fiber 2 g total sugar (1.5 g natural, 0.5 g added) • 220 mg sodium

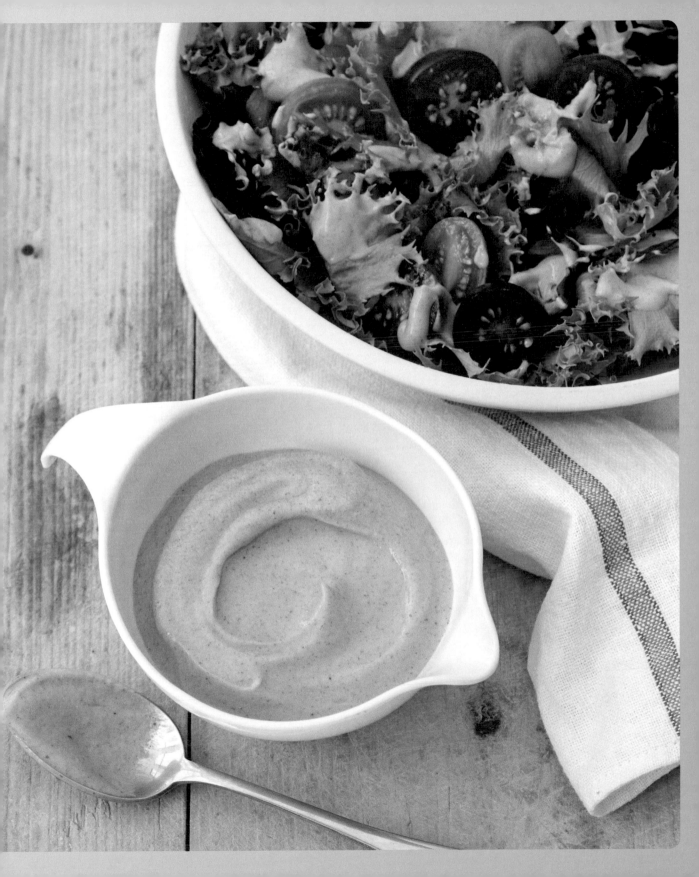

Junk Food

THOUSAND ISLAND DRESSING

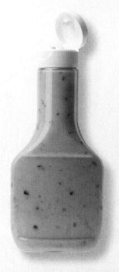

There must be a thousand ways to enjoy this rich and tangy dressing, from salads to sammies . . . even as a dip for veggies or lean protein picks like shrimp. However, the classic combo of mayo and ketchup could easily weigh you down with as many as 150 calories per 2 tablespoons.

My skinny version boasts the classic flavor while still keeping it slim.

Joy Food

THOUSAND ISLAND DRESSING

makes 6 servings

This six-ingredient dressing (that's including salt and pepper) is simple to make and dramatically lighter than your typical store-bought bottle. It's one of my favorite salad toppers, but it also makes a terrific sandwich spread. I hope you'll try it with my health-ified Turkey Reuben (page 78).

½ cup plain nonfat Greek yogurt
2 tablespoons ketchup
2 tablespoons pickle relish or minced pickles
1 teaspoon Worcestershire sauce
¾ teaspoon kosher salt or coarse sea salt
¼ teaspoon ground black pepper

Combine all the ingredients in a small bowl and stir to combine.

---

nutrition information PER 2-TABLESPOON SERVING
18 calories • 2 g protein • 0 g total fat (0 g unsaturated, 0 g saturated) • 0 mg cholesterol • 2.5 g carbs • 0 g fiber 2 g total sugar (0.5 g natural, 1.5 g added) • 285 mg sodium

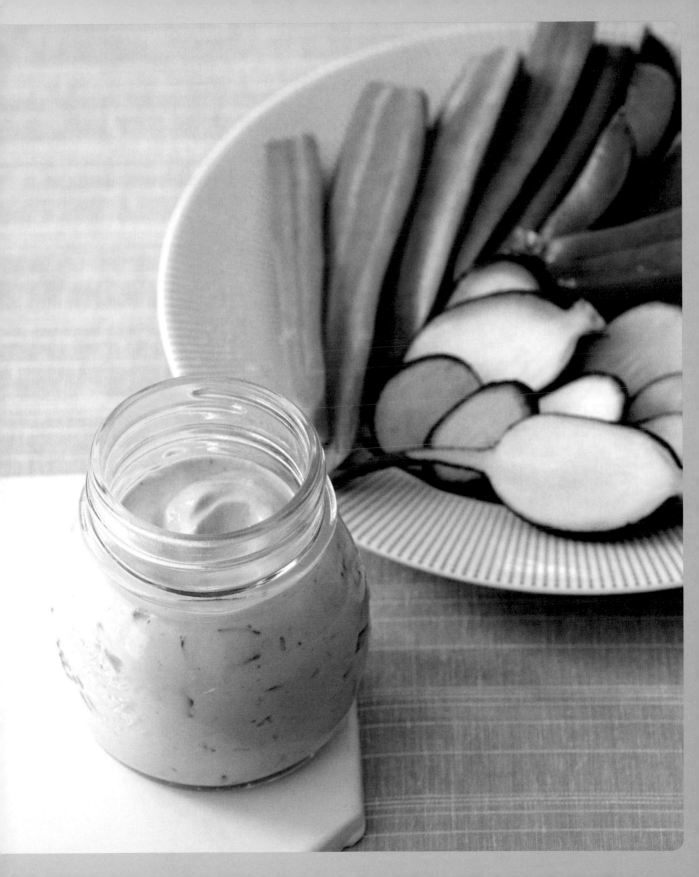

Junk Food

180 CALORIES

CAESAR DRESSING

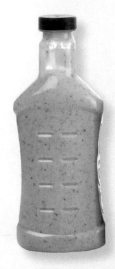

I'm a big fan of creamy Caesar dressing (who isn't?!), but I use it sparingly because it's not exactly the healthiest way to top a salad. Loaded with calories—as many as 180 per 2 tablespoons—it may win the prize for the least diet-friendly way to flavor up your greens. And considering most salads come dressed with 4 to 6 tablespoons, if you were to start a restaurant outing with a Caesar salad appetizer, you're looking at 360 to 540 calories from the dressing alone. Pretty startling.

Build a better salad bowl by using my recipe, with just 40 calories per 2-tablespoon serving of dressing. It's easy to make and even easier to gobble down.

Joy Food

40 CALORIES

CAESAR DRESSING

makes 6 servings

My secret ingredient? Avocado. This creamy produce pick adds a dose of healthy fats and nutrition, while the seasonings flavor it up to perfection. This slim-style dressing beats bottled versions (and homemade calorific creations) any day of the week.

⅓ cup mashed ripe avocado
   (from about ½ an avocado)
1 clove garlic, minced (about 1 teaspoon)
   or ¼ teaspoon garlic powder
2 tablespoons fresh lemon juice
2 teaspoons Worcestershire sauce
½ teaspoon Dijon mustard
¼ cup grated Parmesan cheese
¾ teaspoon kosher salt or coarse sea salt
½ teaspoon ground black pepper
1 teaspoon anchovy paste (optional)

Place all the ingredients plus 6 tablespoons water in a food processor or powerful blender and mix until thoroughly combined and smooth.

---

nutrition information PER 2-TABLESPOON SERVING
40 calories ▪ 2 g protein ▪ 3 g total fat (2 g unsaturated, 1 g saturated) ▪ 0 mg cholesterol ▪ 2 g carbs ▪ 1 g fiber 0 g total sugar (0 g natural, 0 g added) ▪ 234 mg sodium

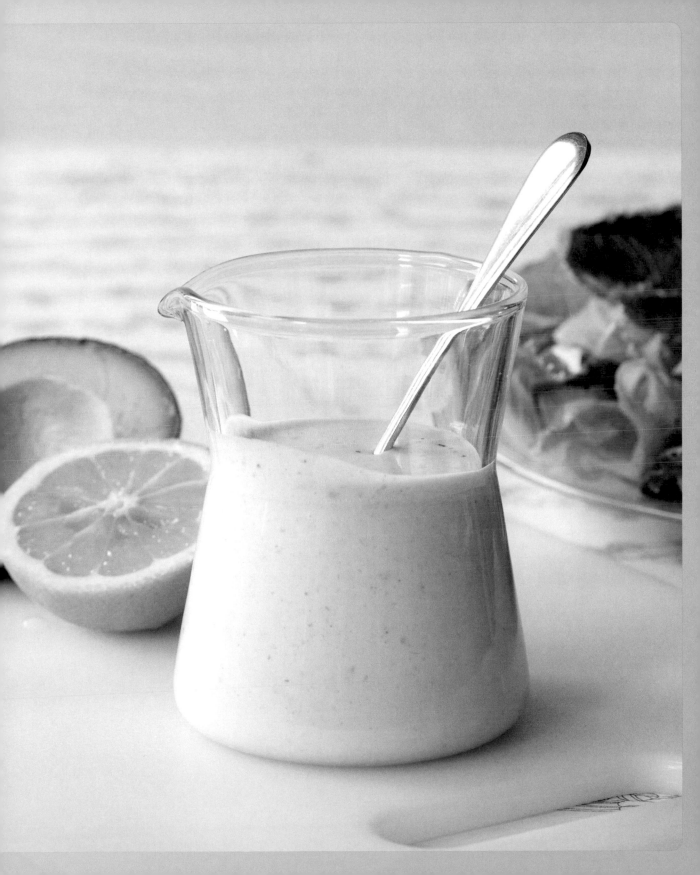

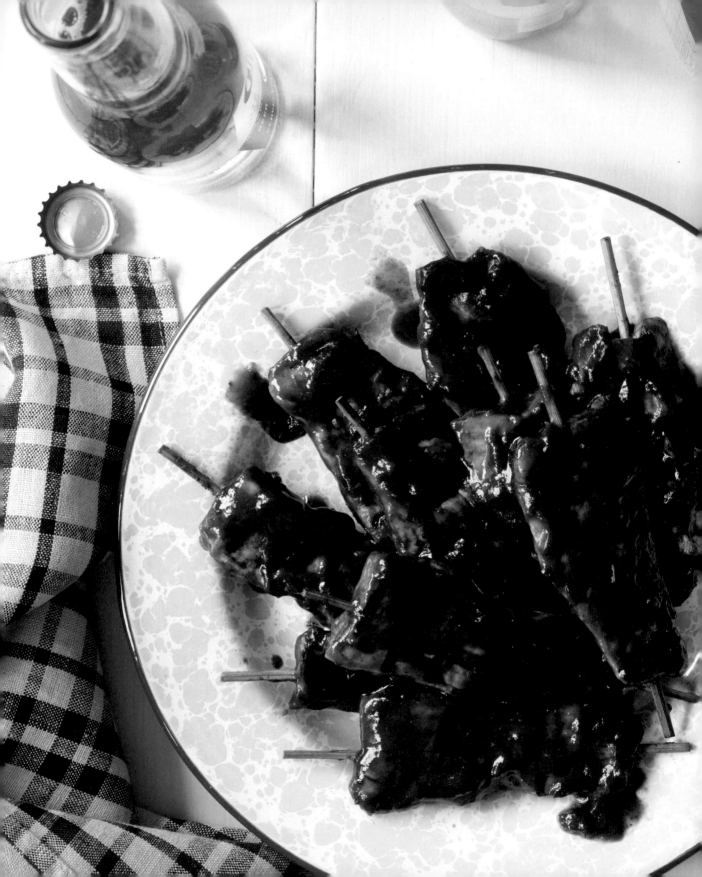

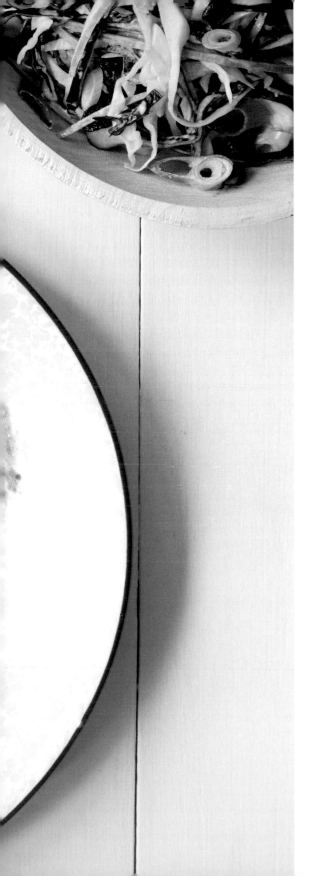

Chapter 5

SIMPLE, SATISFYING SUPPERS

They're the three words that can stop any mom in her tracks and send chills down every dad's spine· "What's for dinner?"

Sometimes, the path of least resistance—picking up the phone and dialing up delivery or spinning through the drive-through—is just so appetizing and seemingly so much easier, especially when time is limited, budget is tight, and palates are picky.

But I have an easy and tasty fix—11 of them, actually. The recipes in this section are tried-and-true renditions of family favorites. They're also low in calories, high in flavor, simple to throw together, and guaranteed hits. You can't go wrong with my chicken Parmesan, barbecue ribs, slow-cooker chili, chicken cacciatore, or turkey tacos. Dinner is served.

Junk Food

1,000 CALORIES

CHICKEN PARM

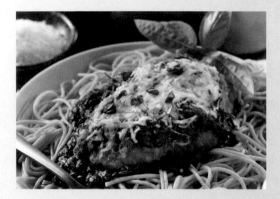

Traditional chicken Parmesan is covered with refined flour and bread crumbs, dunked in a vat of oil for frying, smothered in sauce and cheese, and then served with a pile of starchy pasta. The chicken Parm part alone will run you about 1,000 calories. Pair it with a restaurant-sized portion of pasta, and you're probably looking at 1,400 calories — plus a boatload of saturated fat and salt. In fact, an order from one popular restaurant chain contains 3,000 milligrams of sodium, much more than most people should consume in a day. Yikes!

While classic chicken Parm will never earn health-food status, there's no denying that it's fabulous. And because we're not giving it up anytime soon, here are two great tips to cut about 750 calories at any Italian restaurant, while still enjoying that same delicious flavor:

1. Ask for *grilled* chicken instead of breaded and fried.
2. Request vegetables to be mixed into your pasta.

This strategy works great for dining out, but when you're dining in, whip up my slimmed-down recipe for just 310 calories.

Joy Food

310 CALORIES

GRILLED CHICKEN PARM

makes 4 servings

No need to undo your button or loosen your belt buckle after enjoying my slimming—and totally satisfying—rendition of this classic Italian dish. For far fewer calories and half the prep work, this low-carb, gluten-free entrée will undoubtedly become part of your regular menu rotation. Round it off with some roasted broccoli and the option for whole-grain pasta or brown rice. There's even room for dessert afterward!

> Four 6-ounce boneless, skinless chicken breasts
> ½ cup marinara sauce, homemade or store-bought
> 1 cup shredded part-skim mozzarella cheese
> 4 teaspoons grated Parmesan cheese
> Dried oregano (optional)
> Red pepper flakes (optional)

Grill the chicken breasts or sauté them over medium heat in a skillet coated with nonstick oil spray for 5 to 7 minutes per side, or until they are no longer pink in the center.

Preheat the broiler. Line a baking sheet with aluminum foil and coat the foil with nonstick oil spray.

Transfer the chicken breasts to the prepared baking sheet. Top each chicken breast with 2 tablespoons marinara sauce, ¼ cup mozzarella cheese, 1 teaspoon Parmesan cheese, and a pinch of oregano and red pepper flakes, if desired. Place the chicken under the broiler until the cheese is hot and bubbly (or microwave it for 30 to 60 seconds to melt the cheese).

---

nutrition information PER SERVING
310 calories ▪ 47 g protein ▪ 10.5 g total fat (6.5 g unsaturated, 4 g saturated) ▪ 140 mg cholesterol ▪ 3.5 g carbs ▪ 0 g fiber 1.5 g total sugar (1.5 g natural, 0 g added) ▪ 370 mg sodium

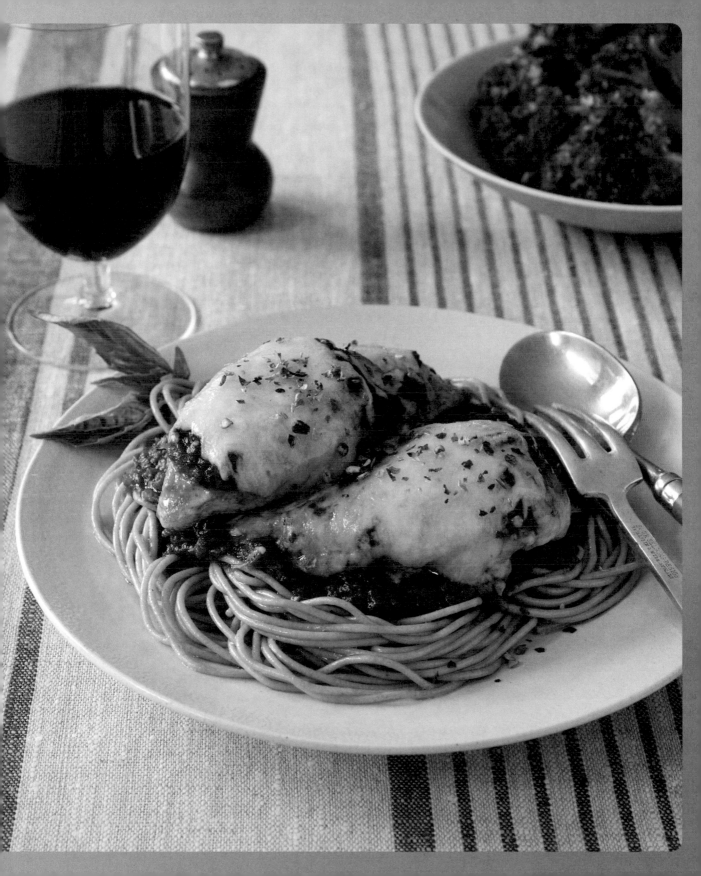

Junk Food

800 CALORIES

CLASSIC CHILI

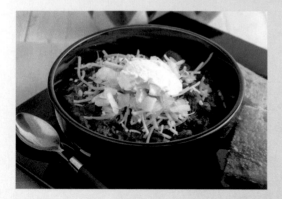

A bowl of chili is the ultimate warm-you-up food, but it can also be fill-you-out fare if you're not careful. While a typical restaurant portion comes packed with nutrient-rich beans, it also delivers fatty meat, calorific cheese, and not-so-skinny sour cream. A standard two-cup serving with classic toppers could easily tally up to 800 calories. To make matters worse, a bowl of chili is traditionally served with fried tortilla chips or a warm roll. Dig in to the entire spread and your diet is toast.

On the flip side, when you're in charge of what goes into—and what stays out of—your pot, the meal can make a 180-degree health turn. Turns out, chili can be harmful or healthful depending on the ingredients.

My husband, Ian, and I are both obsessed with making chili. Sometimes we fight over who gets to cook it. We have tons of fun playing around with creative combos and have made everything from Buffalo Chicken Chili with chopped carrots, celery, and lots of hot sauce . . . to Thai Turkey Chili with peanut butter, soy sauce, and ginger. For this meal makeover, I stuck with a fuss-free, classic recipe. Hope you enjoy it.

Joy Food

345 CALORIES

CLASSIC CHILI
makes 6 servings

There's nothing better than a meal that cooks itself. Take just five minutes to prep, toss all the ingredients in a slow cooker, and a few hours later, enjoy a delicious, healthy, homemade meal. Alternatively, you can follow my directions for the stove-top version. Whichever you choose, the recipe is so simple—it's foolproof. Yet it will look like you slaved for hours in the kitchen. (Shhh! Don't say a word . . . just go with it.)

> Two 28-ounce cans diced tomatoes
> 1¼ pounds ground turkey
>   (at least 90 percent lean)
> 2 red bell peppers, finely chopped
>   (about 2 cups)
> 1 yellow onion, finely chopped
> One 15.5-ounce can pinto beans,
>   drained and rinsed
> One 15.5-ounce can red kidney beans,
>   drained and rinsed
> 2 tablespoons chili powder
> 2 tablespoons cumin
> 2 teaspoons garlic powder
> 2 teaspoons oregano
> ¼ teaspoon cayenne pepper (use ½ teaspoon if
>   you like it hot)
> ¼ teaspoon kosher salt or coarse sea salt

For slow-cooker chili: Drain and discard liquid from both cans of tomatoes, place all the ingredients into a slow cooker (see note), and mix well. Cover and cook the chili on high for 4 hours or on low for 8 hours. When chili is ready, remove lid carefully, stir thoroughly to blend all ingredients and liquid, and ladle into bowls.

Note: If you prefer a chunkier consistency, brown the ground turkey in a skillet coated with nonstick oil spray *before* tossing it in the slow cooker with all the other

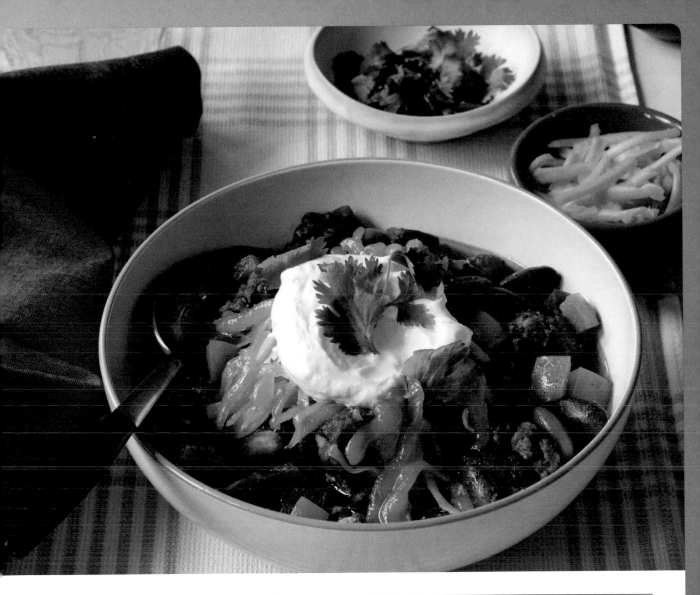

ingredients. While I love the convenience of tossing raw meat into the slow cooker with everything else, it results in a thinner consistency.

For stove-top chili: Brown the turkey in a large Dutch oven or pot coated with nonstick oil spray. Once the turkey is cooked, add the peppers and onion and sauté for 3 to 4 minutes. Drain the liquid from *only one* can of tomatoes, then add the drained tomatoes, the can of undrained tomatoes (including liquid), and all the remaining ingredients to the pot. Stir to combine and simmer for at least 20 minutes or until desired thickness.

Ladle the chili into bowls and enjoy.

nutrition information PER 2-CUP SERVING

345 calories ▪ 29 g protein ▪ 9 g total fat (7 g unsaturated, 2 g saturated) ▪ 65mg cholesterol ▪ 39 g carbs ▪ 13 g fiber 8 g total sugar (8 g natural, 0 g added) ▪ 740 mg sodium

TASTY TWIST Love chili with toppings but don't want a lot of extra calories? Serve each hearty bowl with 2 tablespoons of nonfat plain Greek yogurt (16 calories) or light sour cream (40 calories), 2 tablespoons of shredded reduced-fat cheese (40 calories), and chopped cilantro (0 calories).

Junk Food

SPANISH PAELLA

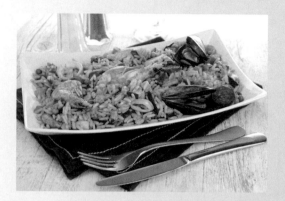

Paella is a traditional Spanish dish that features different protein sources (often meat, chicken, or fish), a variety of veggies (including green beans, peas, and peppers), and wonderful spices like paprika and saffron. It is also starch central, due to the mounds of carb-y rice, and therefore, heavy on calories—as many as 680 per plate.

I lightened it up substantially by making a version using "cauliflower rice." It sounds crazy, but believe me, this trick works. By pulsing the veggie florets in a food processor (or by using a grater), you can create low-carb "rice" out of cauliflower that tastes amazing . . . especially after it soaks up the sauce and seasonings. A hearty 2-cup portion of my paella has fewer than 200 calories. Now, that's a tasty deal.

Joy Food

SPANISH PAELLA

makes 7 servings

I was challenged to build a better paella—slim down the calories and beef up the nutrition—by a viewer of NBC's *Today* show. I revealed this yummy recipe live on the show, and it was a smashing success with my girlfriends Kathie Lee Gifford and Hoda Kotb. In fact, while we were still on the air, they went back for a second (and third) taste! Then, as soon as the segment concluded, the camera crew dove into the bowl, too. Now it's your turn. I think you'll agree it's good to the last bite.

> 1¼ pounds spicy turkey or chicken sausage links
> ½ red bell pepper, finely chopped
> ½ yellow onion, finely chopped
> 1 large head cauliflower
> 2 cloves garlic, minced
> 1 teaspoon red pepper flakes
> 1 teaspoon paprika
> ¼ teaspoon kosher salt or coarse sea salt
> 1½ cups frozen green peas, thawed
> 2 pounds shrimp, peeled and deveined
> Salt and pepper to taste
> Saffron to taste (optional)

Liberally coat a large pot with nonstick oil spray and warm over medium heat. Add the sausages, pepper, and onion.

When the sausages are partially cooked and firm enough to slice (I generally slice them while they're still in the pot), cut them into bite-sized pieces. Stir occasionally, until the sausages are fully cooked.

While the sausages cook, make the cauliflower rice: Rinse the cauliflower and pat it dry (it's important for the cauliflower to be as dry as possible). Break the cauliflower head into large

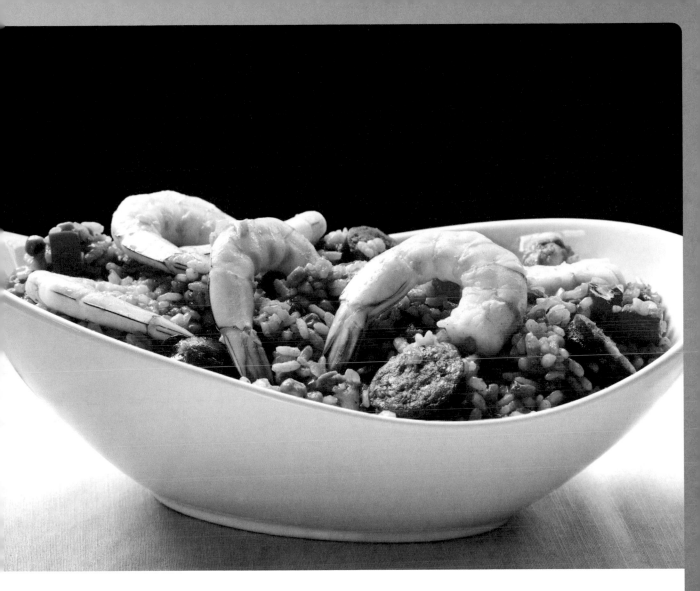

florets. One small batch at a time, place a handful of florets into a food processor and pulse for a few seconds to chop into rice-like pieces. Be careful not to overpulse or load too many florets into the food processor at one time, or you'll wind up with pureed cauliflower.

Transfer each batch of cauliflower rice to a bowl until you finish the entire head. If you don't have a food processor, you can create small, uniform pieces using a coarse grater.

Add the cauliflower rice to the pot with the cooked sausage. Then add the garlic, red pepper flakes, paprika, and salt, sautéing over medium heat for about 15 minutes, scraping the bottom to incorporate the sausage flavors.

Add the peas and shrimp to the pot and mix well. Cover and continue to cook until the shrimp is fully cooked, about 8 to 10 minutes. Add salt and pepper and a pinch of saffron, if desired. Serve and enjoy.

nutrition information PER 2-CUP SERVING
195 calories ▪ 24 g protein ▪ 7 g total fat (7 g unsaturated, 0 g saturated) ▪ 110 mg cholesterol ▪ 8 g carbs ▪ 2 g fiber 2 g total sugar (1.5 g natural, 0.5 g added) ▪ 780 mg sodium

Junk Food

BARBECUE RIBS

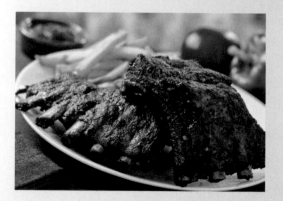

Ready for a barbecue bombshell? As tasty as a juicy rack of barbecue ribs is, it will cost you, on average, 1,200 calories and 70 grams of fat (20 of which are saturated). That's like your arteries' worst nightmare.

In order to health-ify this comfort food fave, I had to get crafty. First, I replaced marbled, fatty rib meat with thinly sliced, lean pork tenderloin. To soak in plenty of flavor, I marinated the meat in a low-sugar barbecue sauce (you can use your favorite brand or make your own), and I used skewers to act like the bones in my recipe. This way you can get down and dirty and eat 'em with your hands—just like regular ribs.

A 10-ounce serving of my "ribs" (the same amount of meat found on a typical rack) contains less than *half* the number of calories of the traditional version—518 calories. And most people will eat a smaller portion, so consider this: 4 ounces of mine are just 207 calories. They are finger-lickin' good!

Joy Food

BARBECUE "RIBS"

makes 6 servings

I totally rethought ribs: I slice lean pork tenderloin, put it on skewers, coat it with barbecue sauce, and pop it on the grill. The result: an amazingly flavorful (and manly!) dish my husband and son cannot get enough of. You can also skip the skewers and prepare boneless "ribs." Test it out on your family, and because it's so light and lean, you can feel free to double up on portions.

> 2 pounds pork tenderloin
> 1 cup barbecue sauce (any brand with no more than 40 calories per 2 tablespoons)
> 6 wood skewers

Slice the pork tenderloin into thin strips that are approximately ¼ inch thick, 4 inches long, and 1½ inches wide.

Add the pork slices and barbecue sauce to a dish or sealable bag and marinate in the refrigerator for at least 2 hours.

Soak skewers in water for about 20 minutes to keep them from burning on the grill.

Preheat the grill or a grill pan to high.

Carefully slide each pork loin slice onto a skewer lengthwise so the meat stays flat and the skewer becomes the "rib."

Place the "ribs" on the hot grill and pour the remaining marinade over the raw meat. Cook for 4 to 6 minutes on each side, or until cooked to desired doneness.

---

nutrition information PER SERVING
208 calories ▪ 33 g protein ▪ 5 g total fat (3.5 g unsaturated, 1.5 g saturated) ▪ 86 mg cholesterol ▪ 8 g carbs ▪ 0 g fiber
5 g total sugar (2.5 g natural, 2.5 g added) ▪ 660 mg sodium

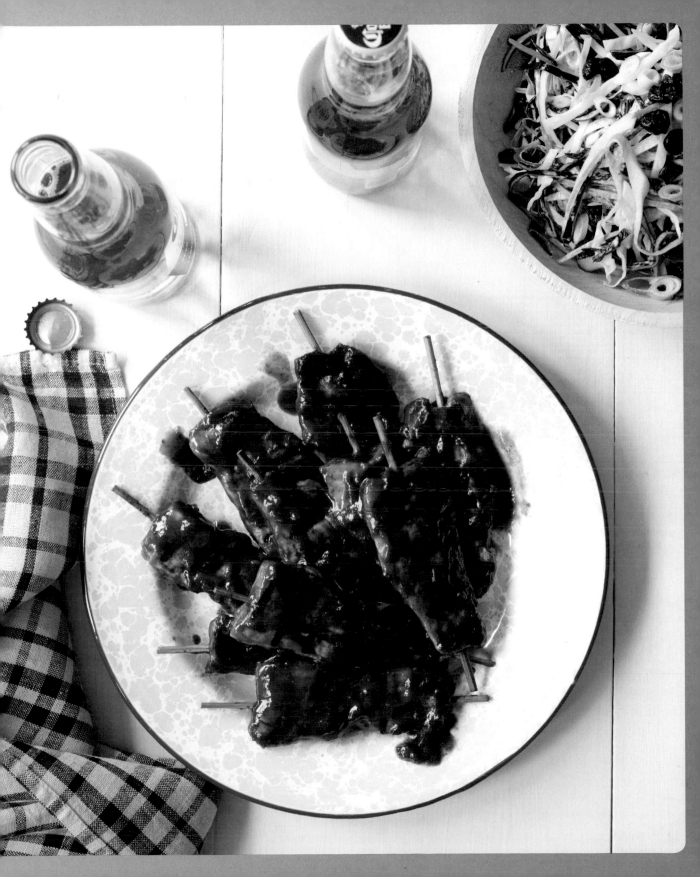

Junk Food

720 CALORIES

TACOS

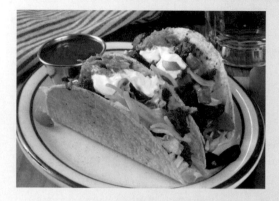

In the mood for Mexican tonight? Get ready to tally the calories and loosen your belt, thanks to all the irresistible ingredients, like seasoned beef, cheese, sour cream, and guacamole (healthy, yes, but also caloric). Check this out: two standard tacos weigh in at about 720 calories . . . eat a third and you're at 1,080. That's one fattening fiesta.

Instead, you can easily make them at home using light and lean ingredients. Check out my slim spin, which is equally fabulous and filling—*muy bueno!*

Joy Food

370 CALORIES

TURKEY TACOS
makes 4 servings

In my house, Turkey Tacos are a sure thing. They're even a hit with my kids' picky-eater friends. And nobody has ever suspected the healthy swaps: lean ground turkey, reduced-fat cheese, and colorful, chopped veggies. For a few extra calories, feel free to elaborate on my ingredient list and add small bowls filled with chopped bell pepper, red onion, beans, and corn. To make dinner even more memorable, set up a toppings bar. This way, everyone has fun building their favorite combos.

1¼ pounds ground turkey (at least 90 percent lean)
1 packet taco seasoning mix, preferably low-sodium
2 cups chopped or shredded lettuce
1 large tomato, chopped
1 cup shredded reduced-fat cheddar
   or Mexican-blend cheese
8 corn taco shells, hard or soft
Salsa and/or hot sauce (optional)
Nonfat plain Greek yogurt or light sour cream
   (optional)

In a large skillet misted with nonstick oil spray, cook the turkey over medium-high heat until browned. Drain the fat. Stir in the taco seasoning and water (as indicated on the seasoning package) and bring the mixture to a boil. Reduce the heat to medium-low and simmer, stirring occasionally, until nearly all the liquid has evaporated, 5 to 6 minutes.

Evenly divide the turkey mixture, lettuce, tomato, and cheese among the taco shells. Top with salsa, hot sauce, and Greek yogurt, if desired. Alternatively, set up a toppings bar and let everyone fend for themselves.

nutrition information PER SERVING OF 2 TACOS
370 calories ▪ 43 g protein ▪ 13 g total fat (5 g saturated, 8 g unsaturated) ▪ 94 mg cholesterol ▪ 22 g carbs ▪ 2 g fiber
1 g total sugar (1 g natural, 0 g added) ▪ 850 mg sodium

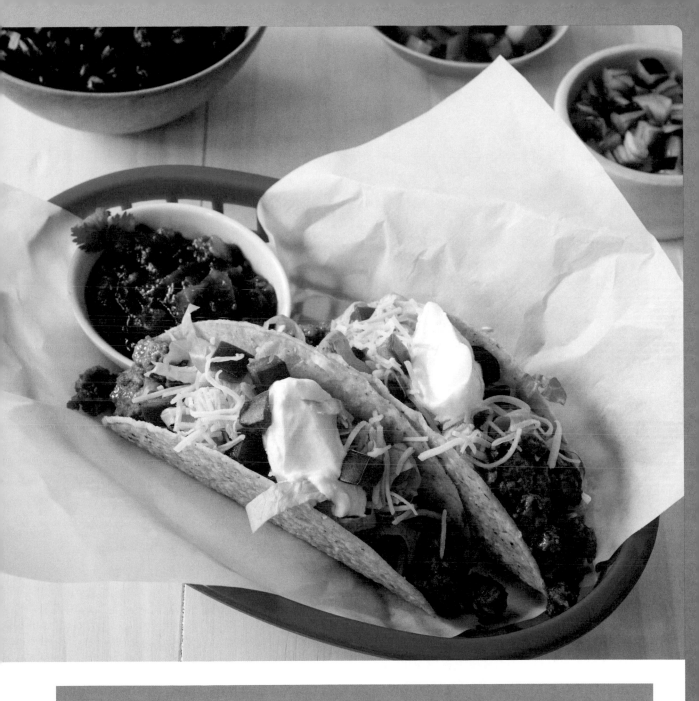

TASTY TWIST Serve your tacos with my simple Seasoned Black Beans! Sauté 1 chopped yellow onion in a saucepan coated with nonstick oil spray over medium heat until soft and browned, about 8 minutes. Add one 15-ounce can of black beans (rinsed and drained), 1 teaspoon cumin, 1 teaspoon garlic powder, and 1 teaspoon Dijon mustard, and sauté over medium-high heat for about 5 minutes. Season with salt and pepper to taste. Makes 4 (½-cup) servings. Each serving contains 110 calories, 7 g protein, and 8 g fiber.

Junk Food

1,100 CALORIES

BACON CHEESEBURGER

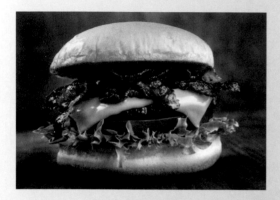

Order up a bacon cheeseburger from a local burger joint and you could easily chow down the majority of a day's worth of calories, while exceeding your artery-clogging fat limit by a landslide. And that's not even including the greasy, salty side of fries. Let's just say the combo is not conducive to happy times at your next physical or beach party.

Instead, prepare your burger at home with a few simple swaps: fatty beef patty out, lean poultry patty in; pork bacon out, turkey bacon in; full-fat cheese out, reduced-fat in. The new and improved version is just 425 calories and just as filling and flavorful. You'll see.

> **CHOOSE IT TO LOSE IT** Trade in your bacon cheeseburger twice a week and, in a year's time, you'll save at least 70,000 calories and could drop about 20 pounds.

Joy Food

425 CALORIES

BACON CHEESEBURGER

makes 4 servings

Every burger lover needs a simple, good-for-you recipe they can call on whenever a craving strikes. This is my personal go-to creation, and when it's coupled with Sweet Potato Fries (page 100), it's (burger) heaven on earth. Follow my exact directions, or simply use them for inspiration to make your own delicious variation. For example, you can swap ground turkey for ground sirloin or bison and pile on sautéed mushrooms and caramelized onions. You can't go wrong.

1 pound ground turkey
   (at least 90 percent lean)
¼ cup ketchup
1 tablespoon spicy brown mustard
1 teaspoon garlic powder
1 chopped onion (optional)
4 slices turkey bacon
4 slices reduced-fat cheese, any variety
4 whole-grain hamburger buns
Lettuce, tomatoes, onions, pickles, ketchup,
   mustard (optional)

Combine the turkey, ketchup, mustard, garlic powder, and onion, if desired, in a small bowl. Divide the mixture into 4 equal-sized portions and shape them into burgers. Set aside.

Coat a skillet with nonstick oil spray and warm it over medium heat. Add the turkey bacon and cook until crispy, following package directions. Set the bacon aside on a paper towel to drain.

Reapply nonstick oil spray to the skillet and cook the turkey burgers about 5 minutes per side. When the burgers are done, top each with 1 slice of cheese.

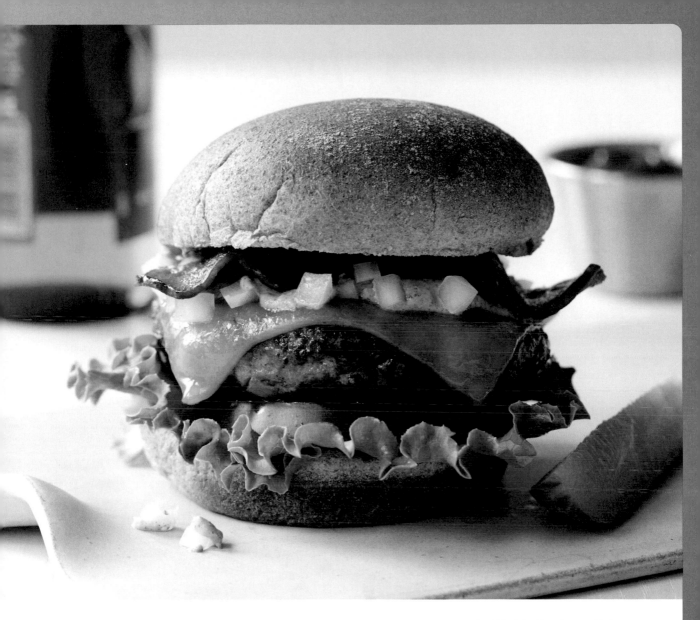

Cover the skillet to allow the cheese to melt.

Toast the bun.

Once the cheese has melted, place each cheeseburger on a toasted bottom bun, and add 1 slice of cooked turkey bacon (split into two piecies) on top.

Layer each with lettuce, tomato, onions, pickles, and a squirt of ketchup or mustard, if desired. Add the top bun and dig in.

nutrition information PER SERVING

425 calories ▪ 36 g protein ▪ 17 g total fat (6 g saturated fat, 11 g unsaturated fat) ▪ 115 mg cholesterol ▪ 28 g carbs 3 g fiber ▪ 6 g total sugar (3.5 natural, 2.5 added) ▪ 770 mg sodium

TASTY TWIST Pile your burger with flavorful add-ons like lettuce, tomato, onion, and sliced avocado. Need a low-cal special sauce? Try my "metchup," made by mixing low-fat mayo with ketchup.

Junk Food

420 CALORIES

SHEPHERD'S PIE

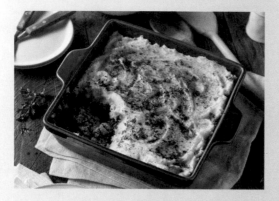

Meat pie with a mashed-potato crust? Not surprisingly, this is no diet dish. But if you're a meat-and-potato fanatic, you'll be happy to hear that I've mastered a healthier version without sacrificing any of the deliciousness.

This recipe redo was born when I was invited to a neighbor's potluck dinner party. Knowing that you can't go wrong showing up with a meat-and-potato casserole, I took a valiant stab at a skinnier—yet just as hearty—version of this classic. I left with an empty serving dish, and woke up the next morning to find several e-mails asking for the recipe. It was a winner.

Joy Food

174 CALORIES

SHEPHERD'S PIE

makes 9 servings

Love warm and comforting shepherd's pie? Me, too. You and your family can enjoy it as often as you like with my tasty take on the beloved English classic. All you need are two quick and easy calorie-cutting tricks: swap ground beef for lean ground turkey and replace regular mashed potatoes with mashed cauliflower. Voilà—a thinner dinner!

MASHED CAULIFLOWER TOPPING

2 heads cauliflower, cut into medium florets (about 6 cups)

4 cloves garlic, peeled, or 1 teaspoon garlic powder

¼ cup light or reduced-fat cream cheese

1 teaspoon kosher salt or coarse sea salt

½ teaspoon ground black pepper

⅓ cup shredded reduced-fat sharp cheddar cheese

MEAT FILLING

1 onion, finely chopped

2 carrots, finely chopped

2 ribs celery, finely chopped

½ pound button mushrooms, quartered or halved

2 cloves garlic, minced, or ½ teaspoon garlic powder

1 teaspoon kosher salt or coarse sea salt

½ teaspoon ground black pepper

1 pound ground turkey breast (at least 90 percent lean)

2 teaspoons chopped rosemary leaves or ¾ teaspoon dried rosemary

½ teaspoon chopped thyme leaves or ½ teaspoon dried thyme

2 teaspoons tomato paste

1 teaspoon Worcestershire sauce

2 tablespoons flour

1 cup low-sodium chicken broth

1 cup fresh, frozen, or canned corn kernels

1¼ cups fresh, frozen, or canned peas

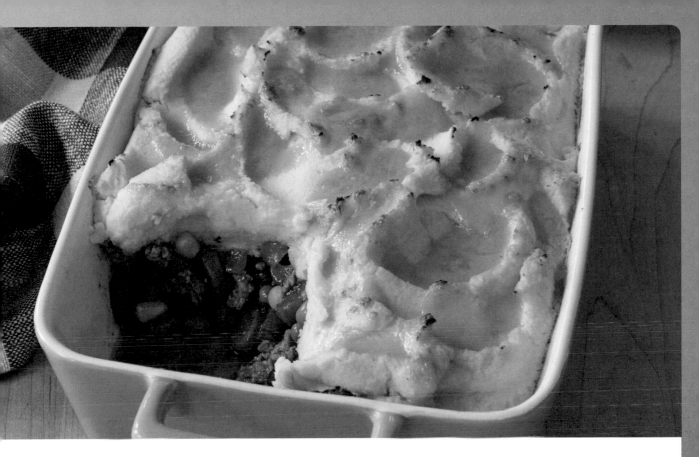

To make the mashed cauliflower, steam the cauliflower in a large covered pot with minimal water until it's fork-tender, about 20 minutes. Drain the cauliflower thoroughly in a colander, and return it to the pot over medium-low heat. Mash the cauliflower with a fork or potato masher.

Add the garlic, cream cheese, salt, and pepper and continue stirring until everything is well blended. Note: Using an immersion blender will help create a creamy, mashed potato–like consistency. Remove from the heat and set aside.

To make the meat filling, liberally coat an extra-large skillet or Dutch oven with nonstick oil spray and warm over medium heat. Add the onion, carrots, celery, mushrooms, and garlic to the pan, season with the salt and pepper, and cook until the onions are translucent and the vegetables are soft, 10 to 15 minutes.

Add the turkey to the pan with the vegetables and cook for about 5 minutes over medium-high heat,

gently breaking up the turkey. Add the rosemary, thyme, tomato paste, and Worcestershire sauce, and cook, stirring, until the tomato paste dissolves, 1 to 2 minutes.

Add the flour and stir until you can no longer see it, about 1 minute. Add the chicken broth and cook, stirring, until it thickens, 1 to 2 minutes. Add the corn and peas and stir to combine.

Preheat the oven to 400°F.

Pour the filling into a 9 x 13–inch baking dish, spreading it into an even layer. Top the filling with the mashed cauliflower, spreading it into an even layer. Sprinkle the cheddar cheese on top, and bake for 20 minutes or until the cheese melts and begins to brown.

nutrition information PER SERVING
174 calories • 16 g protein • 7 g total fat (5 g unsaturated, 2 g saturated) • 43 mg cholesterol • 15 g carbs • 4 g fiber 5 g total sugar (5 g natural, 0 g added) • 415 mg sodium

Junk Food

CHICKEN CACCIATORE

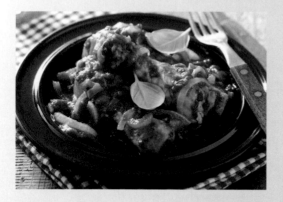

Chicken cacciatore is an Italian classic that's generally made by coating dark meat chicken (thighs, wings, and/or drumsticks with the skin on) in flour, sautéing them in oil with vegetables, and then dousing everything in a tasty red sauce. It's great for flavor, but the chicken skin and excessive oil push the calories unnecessarily high.

My version uses skinless chicken breasts flavored with plenty of peppers, onions, and mushrooms. I cook the entire thing in one pot in less than an hour. Easiest. Recipe. Ever.

Joy Food

CHICKEN CACCIATORE

makes 6 servings

Most cuisines have a hunter's stew—a slow-cooked meal where favorite meats, vegetables, and seasonings come together in one pot. This one is my easy-peasy take on Italy's famed cacciatore. It's made with lean chicken breast and sautéed vegetables simmered in flavorful marinara sauce. Feel free to swap in whatever veggies you love most, and if you want some extra pizazz, finish it off with a splash of balsamic vinegar. Trust me, no one will leave the table hungry—it's family-friendly and deliciously filling.

1½ pounds boneless, skinless chicken breast, cut into 2-inch chunks
¼ teaspoon kosher salt or coarse sea salt
¼ teaspoon ground black pepper
3 cloves garlic, minced, or ¾ teaspoon garlic powder
1 yellow onion, thinly sliced
2 bell peppers, thinly sliced
One 10-ounce package button mushrooms, sliced
One 24-ounce jar marinara sauce, store-bought or homemade
1 tablespoon aged balsamic vinegar (optional)

Liberally coat a large pot or Dutch oven with nonstick oil spray and warm it over medium-high heat. Season the chicken with the salt and pepper. Add the chicken to the pot and cook it until it is slightly browned on all sides, 5 to 7 minutes. Transfer the chicken to a plate and set aside.

Reapply nonstick oil spray to the pot and add the garlic, onion, peppers, and mushrooms, and sauté until soft, about 7 minutes. Drain the excess liquid.

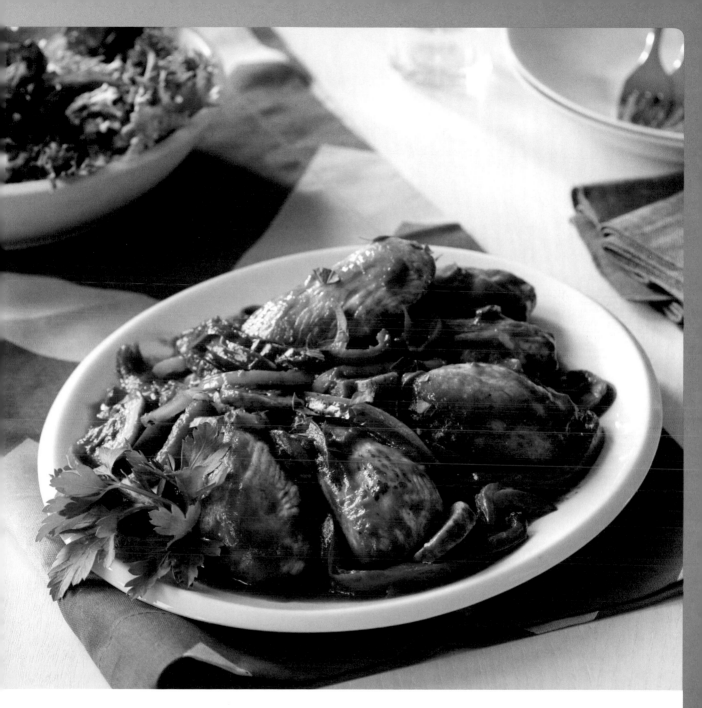

Add the cooked chicken and marinara sauce to the pot with the veggies, and mix thoroughly. Reduce the heat to low, cover the pot, and simmer for 30 minutes.

Uncover the pot, stir, and continue to simmer for an additional 10 minutes. Stir in the balsamic vinegar, if desired, just before serving.

nutrition information PER SERVING

195 calories ▪ 27 g protein ▪ 3.5 g total fat (3 g unsaturated, 0.5 g saturated) ▪ 73 mg cholesterol ▪ 15 g carbs ▪ 3 g fiber 7.5 g total sugar (7.5 g natural, 0 g added) ▪ 565 mg sodium

Junk Food

CHICKEN ENCHILADAS

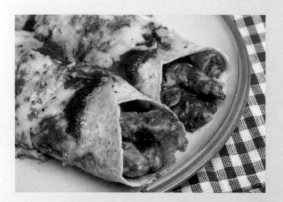

Welcome to Mexican mayhem. Let's just say that when you enjoy a couple of enchiladas, the corn tortilla isn't the only thing that's going to be stuffed. The delicious south-of-the-border dish involves filling the tortilla with a variety of ingredients, including chicken, cheese, veggies, and more, and then topping it with even more cheese and a spicy chili sauce. Mouthwatering, but not waist-friendly at 600 calories per serving (that's two small enchiladas without sides). A standard order at popular Mexican restaurants with the customary rice and beans on the side will cost you north of the (1,000-calorie) border.

I make a super-slimming version with pulled chicken in the slow cooker. It comes together quickly and is always a hit with my family and our ever-expanding guest list.

Joy Food

CHICKEN ENCHILADAS

makes 8 servings

My simple pulled-chicken recipe couldn't be any easier and gives ordinary enchiladas an amazing shot of flavor—you can enjoy two for only 315 calories. I toss all of the chicken fixin's into my slow cooker in the A.M. before leaving for work. When I come home later in the day, I quickly assemble the enchiladas and pop them in the oven. Dinner is served in less than 20 minutes, and my family *flips out* for this indulgent Mexican classic.

PULLED-CHICKEN FILLING
1½ pounds boneless, skinless chicken breasts
½ cup salsa, homemade or store-bought
1 teaspoon garlic powder
½ onion, finely chopped
2 teaspoons taco seasoning

ENCHILADAS
2 cups enchilada or taco sauce, homemade
  or store-bought
2 cups shredded reduced-fat
  Mexican-blend cheese
16 small tortillas (corn or flour)

To make the pulled-chicken filling, add all the ingredients to a slow cooker and set on high for 4 hours or low for 8 hours. When the chicken is done (you'll notice a large amount of liquid in the slow cooker; this is normal), shred it with a fork until all of the liquid within the slow cooker is incorporated.

To make the enchiladas, preheat the oven to 350°F. Coat the bottom of two 9 x 13–inch baking pans with a thin layer of the enchilada sauce.

Microwave the tortillas for about 30 seconds to make them warm and flexible. Place one tortilla at a time on

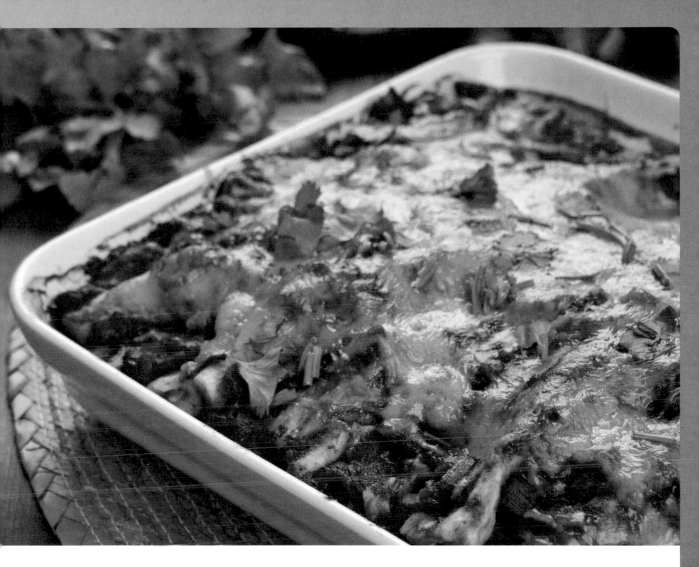

the prepared pan, spreading 1 heaping tablespoon of enchilada sauce evenly over the top of each, adding ¼ cup pulled chicken, and rolling it up. Place the fold sides of the enchiladas underneath, to keep the enchiladas from unraveling. Repeat this process with the remaining tortillas and filling.

Once all the enchiladas are set, spread the remaining enchilada sauce over the top, and sprinkle on the cheese. Place in the oven for about 15 minutes, until the cheese is hot and bubbly.

---

nutrition information PER SERVING OF 2 ENCHILADAS
315 calories • 28 g protein • 10.5 g total fat (6.5 g unsaturated, 4 g saturated) • 70 mg cholesterol • 29 g carbs • 3 g fiber 1 g total sugar (1 g natural, 0 g added) • 843 mg sodium

> **TASTY TWIST** To heighten the flavor, add a dash of cumin, cayenne pepper, red pepper flakes, or any other preferred seasonings on top of the cheese. Serve the enchiladas with chopped tomatoes, cilantro, scallions, salsa, light sour cream, or nonfat plain Greek yogurt.

Junk Food

GENERAL TSO'S CHICKEN

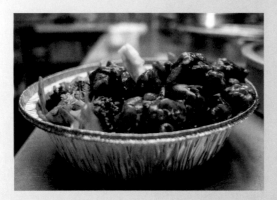

I don't know who General Tso was, but he sure had great taste in chicken. Unfortunately, I don't think he was all too concerned with nutrition: an order of the batter-fried chicken doused in thick sauce will run you about 1,000 calories as well as more than a day's worth of sodium.

When creating my version, I decided to skip the breading and frying and use marinated, sautéed chicken instead. This small tweak provides a big payoff. Then, I focused my efforts on the sauce—because that's what really makes this entrée stand out. Now you can enjoy this flavorful and diet-friendly dish as often as you'd like. Grab your chopsticks!

> **CHOOSE IT TO LOSE IT** Make this substitution once a week and you'll save 39,000 calories at the end of the year, which could translate to 11 pounds lost.

Joy Food

260 CALORIES

GENERAL JOY'S CHICKEN

makes 4 servings

Craving Chinese? Skip the calorie-laden, sodium-packed General Tso's chicken from your local Chinese joint, and whip up my slim-style version instead. I knew I'd struck gold with this recipe when I served it for dinner and my youngest daughter, Ayden Jane, called first dibs on leftovers for lunch. (Happy dance!) The dish has now earned a regular spot in my menu rotation. Make it tonight . . . your fortune says: no regret and lots of compliments.

MARINATED CHICKEN

1 egg white
2 tablespoons reduced-sodium soy sauce
2 tablespoons Chinese rice wine or dry sherry
1½ pounds boneless, skinless chicken breasts, cut into 1-inch cubes

SAUCE

¾ cup 100% no-sugar-added pineapple juice
3 tablespoons reduced-sodium soy sauce
1 tablespoon Chinese rice wine or dry sherry
3 tablespoons low-sodium chicken broth
1 teaspoon toasted sesame oil
¾ teaspoon garlic powder
¾ teaspoon ginger
¼ teaspoon red pepper flakes
1 tablespoon cornstarch or arrowroot flour (see note)
6 scallions (green onions), white and light green parts thinly sliced
1 tablespoon sesame seeds (optional)

To make the marinade, whisk the egg white with the soy sauce and rice wine in a medium bowl. Add the chicken and stir so the marinade evenly coats each piece. Cover the bowl with plastic wrap (or place in

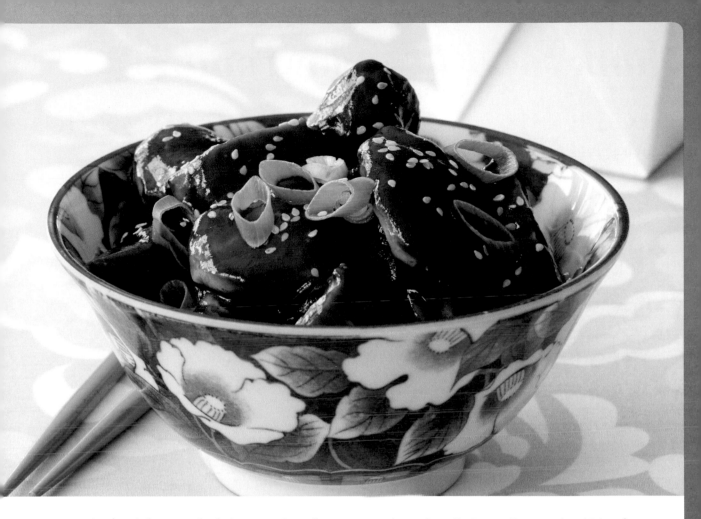

zip-top bag) and place it in the fridge to marinate for at least 30 minutes, or overnight.

To make the sauce, heat the pineapple juice in a small pan over high heat until it comes to a boil. Reduce the heat to low and simmer the juice until it reduces to about ¼ cup and has thickened. This should take about 7 minutes. Remove the pan from the heat and let it cool for a couple of minutes.

Mix the soy sauce, rice wine, chicken broth, sesame oil, garlic powder, ginger, red pepper flakes, and cornstarch in a small bowl. Whisk together so the cornstarch is incorporated and there are no lumps. Set aside.

Spray a large skillet with nonstick oil spray. Pour the chicken and leftover marinade into the skillet and cook over medium-high heat until the chicken pieces are done, about 7 minutes. Remove the chicken from the skillet, cover it to keep it warm, and set it aside.

Pour the sauce mixture into the skillet and cook until the sauce thickens, about 1 minute. Add the cooked chicken to the pan and toss to coat evenly with the sauce. Cook for another 2 minutes, stirring continuously, until the sauce thickens. Garnish with the scallions and sesame seeds, if desired, and serve immediately.

Note: Arrowroot flour can go by many names, including arrowroot, arrowroot starch, arrowroot powder, and ground arrowroot. Don't worry; they're all the same.

---

nutrition information PER SERVING
260 calories ▪ 36 g protein ▪ 6.5 g total fat (5.5 g unsaturated, 1 g saturated) ▪ 105 mg cholesterol ▪ 15 g carbs ▪ 0.5 g fiber 8 g total sugar (8 g natural, 0 g added) ▪ 790 mg sodium

Junk Food

1,040 CALORIES

EGGPLANT PARMESAN

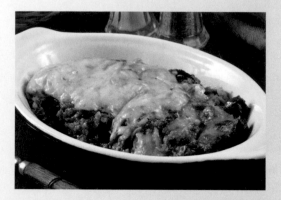

You may think that Eggplant Parmesan is off limits when you're watching your waistline. After all, a plate of this deep-fried delight can easily top 1,040 calories and 54 grams of fat. That's a lot for a vegetable-based entrée.

But here's some eggplant excitement: It turns out, you can enjoy my slim-style version for fewer than 50 calories per slice (nope, not a typo). In fact, you can devour a serving of four slices for a fraction of the original.

Joy Food

192 CALORIES

EGGPLANT PARMESAN

makes 3 servings

Delicious, cheesy, and low in calories, this dish is a game changer. By omitting a few ingredients and tweaking the prep method, I've managed to dramatically cut back on calories, carbs, fat, and salt without sacrificing any of the rich, Italian flavors. Go ahead and whip up a batch for dinner—or for an upcoming party appetizer—and I guarantee you will make it again and again.

> 1 large eggplant
> Salt and pepper to taste
> ¾ cup marinara sauce, store-bought or homemade
> ¾ cup shredded part-skim mozzarella cheese
> ¼ cup grated Parmesan cheese
> Dried oregano to taste
> Red pepper flakes to taste

Preheat the oven to 400°F. Liberally coat a baking sheet with nonstick oil spray and set aside.

Cut off and discard both ends of the eggplant, and then slice the eggplant into rounds (about 12 slices). Arrange the eggplant slices in a single layer on the prepared baking sheet.

Mist the tops of the eggplant slices liberally with nonstick oil spray, and lightly sprinkle with salt and pepper. Bake for 20 minutes, or until the eggplant is soft and golden brown.

Top each slice with about 1 tablespoon marinara sauce and 1 heaping tablespoon mozzarella cheese. Sprinkle the slices with the Parmesan cheese, oregano, and red pepper flakes. Bake for another 5 to 10 minutes, or until the cheese is hot and bubbly.

---

nutrition information PER 4-SLICE SERVING
192 calories ▪ 13 g protein ▪ 8 g total fat (3.5 g unsaturated, 4.5 g saturated) ▪ 23 mg cholesterol ▪ 17 g carbs ▪ 6.5 g fiber 9 g total sugar (9 g natural, 0 g added) ▪ 470 mg sodium

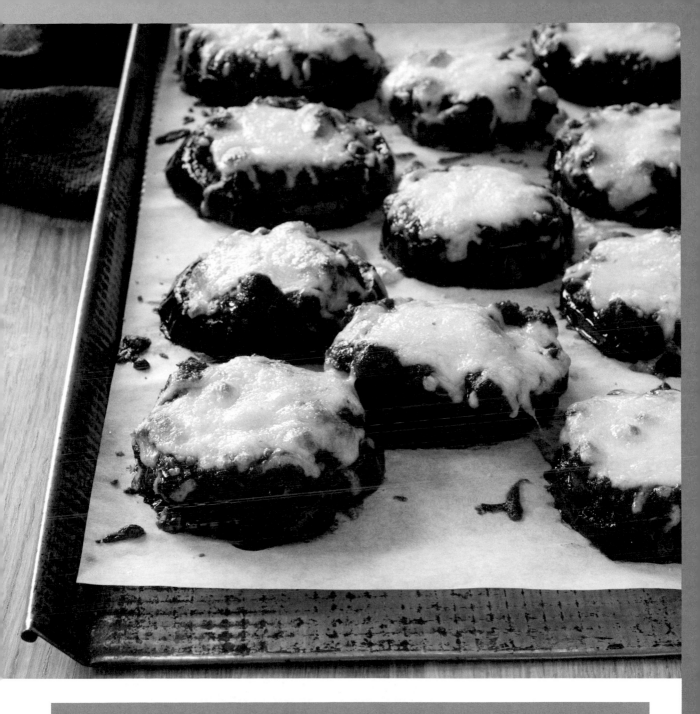

TASTY TWIST Try these tasty Eggplant Parmesan Cabbage Cups: Mix together 2½ cups peeled and diced eggplant, one 28-ounce can crushed tomatoes, ¼ cup shredded part-skim mozzarella, and 2 tablespoons grated Parmesan cheese. Pour the mixture into a baking pan. Sprinkle 2 tablespoons bread crumbs on top, and bake for 30 minutes at 400°F. Scoop 1 tablespoon of the eggplant mixture onto separate cabbage leaves. Garnish with minced parsley. Enjoy 4 cabbage cups for 63 calories.

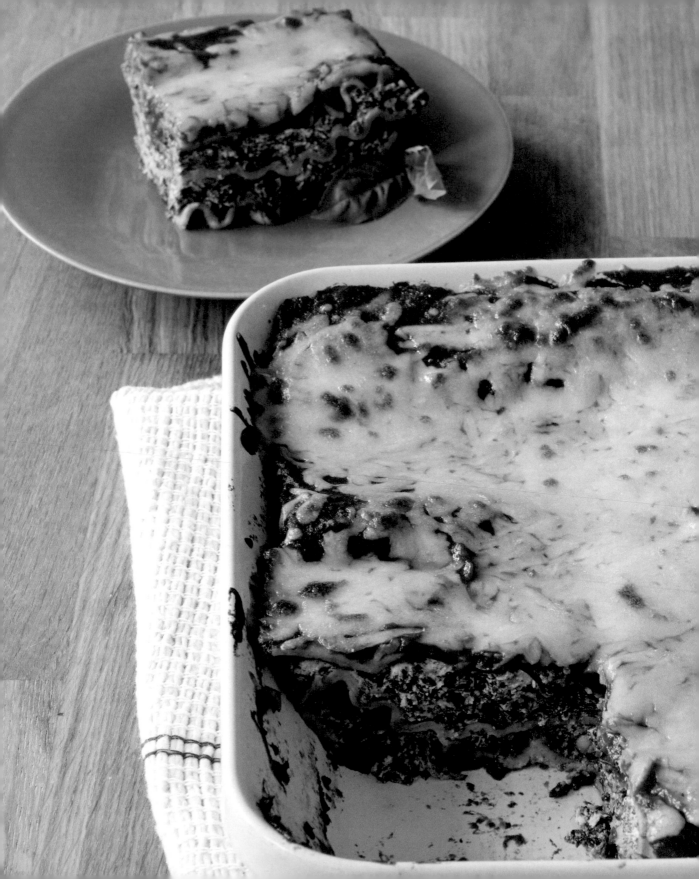

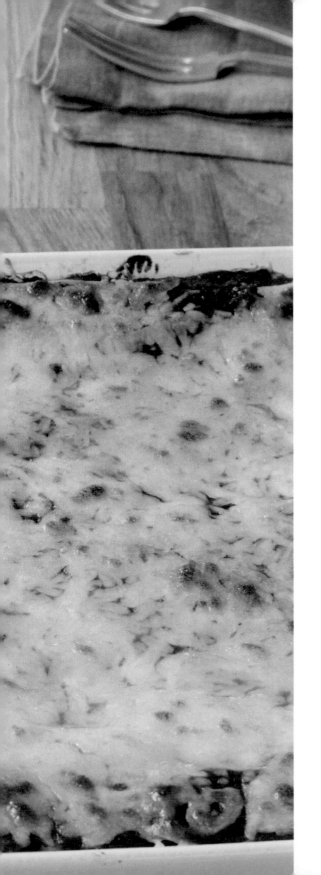

Chapter 6

PALATE-PLEASING PIZZAS AND PASTAS

Whether you're savoring a slice of pizza or tucking into a hearty helping of lasagna, you're sure to enjoy the hallmarks of beloved Italian food: cheesy, comforting, and oh-so-calorific.

Fortunately, you don't have to say so long to spaghetti and meatballs . . . or farewell to fettuccine Alfredo. You can still enjoy classic Italian cuisine with my creative spins on these normally indulgent dishes. Get ready to dig in without guilt or regret. *Mangia!*

Junk Food

500 CALORIES

CHEESE PIZZA

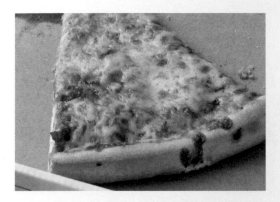

No matter which way you slice it, typical pizzeria pizza is going to cost you—about 500 calories for a large New York–style cheese slice (Hey, here in New York, we like our pizza *big*) or two small slices from a restaurant chain. This is before you consider any of the fattening toppers like sausage, pepperoni, meatballs, or extra cheese. And you know most people don't stop at just one serving.

Here's a slim solution: my Tortilla Pizza. It has just 172 calories for the whole personal pie. Seriously. You can eat the entire thing . . . and go back for seconds, if you're still hungry! Plus, it's so easy to make, and you can personalize it by adding your favorite veggies to pump up the fiber and nutrition. Pizz-a-heaven.

> **CHOOSE IT TO LOSE IT** Swap your slice a few times each week and you'll save more than 34,000 calories annually, which could lead to a loss of 10 pounds at the end of the year.

Joy Food

172 CALORIES

TORTILLA PIZZA
makes 1 serving

Instead of dialing up delivery, try this tasty (and incredibly simple) homemade pizza. It takes minutes to toss together and multitasks as a satisfying after-school snack or healthy dinner coupled with a salad. Amp up the fun by making it a pizza party—let each member of the family pick his or her own toppings.

SAUCE
2 heaping tablespoons tomato sauce
  or favorite marinara sauce
Pinch of oregano
Pinch of garlic powder
Pinch of onion powder

PIZZA
1 large whole-grain or low-carb tortilla
  (any brand with no more than 80 calories
  per tortilla)
¼ cup shredded part-skim mozzarella cheese
Red pepper flakes (optional)
Oregano (optional)
1 teaspoon fresh basil, minced

To make the sauce, mix all the ingredients together in a small bowl. Set aside.

Set the oven to broil.

To make the pizza, place the tortilla on a baking sheet lined with aluminum foil and put it in the oven on the top rack. Cook for about 4 minutes total, flipping after each minute. (Note: Ovens will vary, so watch carefully so the tortilla doesn't burn.)

Remove the tortilla from the oven and spread the sauce on top, covering the majority of the tortilla except for a border of about ¼ inch all the way around.

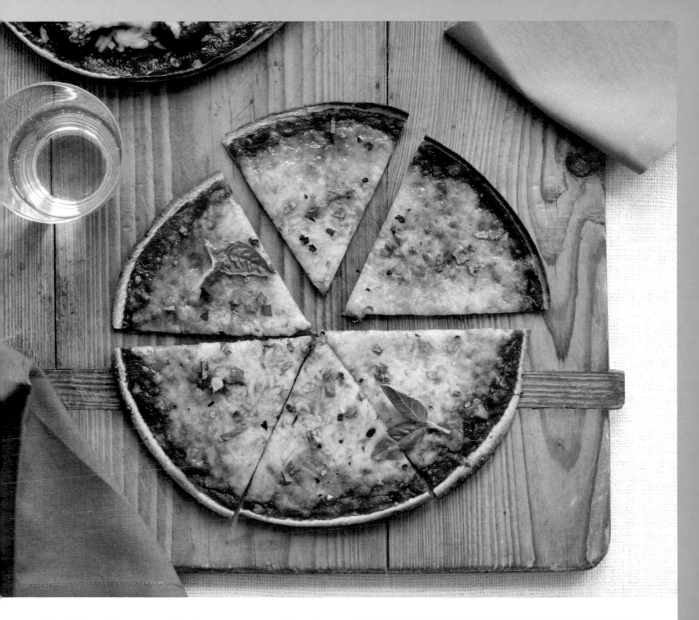

Sprinkle on the mozzarella cheese, season with red pepper flakes and oregano, if desired, and place it back in the oven under the broiler for 30 to 45 seconds, until the cheese is melted.

Garnish with fresh basil. Cut into 4 slices and enjoy your personal pie.

nutrition information PER SERVING
172 calories ▪ 15 g protein ▪ 7.5 g total fat (4.5 g unsaturated, 3 g saturated) ▪ 15 mg cholesterol ▪ 23 g carbs ▪ 6 g fiber 3 g total sugar (3 g natural, 0 g added) ▪ 480 mg sodium

TASTY TWIST Try my Mini English Muffin Pizza. To make, split and toast one whole-grain English muffin, and on each half, add 2 tablespoons each of marinara sauce and part-skim shredded mozzarella cheese. Top with fresh or sautéed veggies. Sprinkle on your preferred seasonings and pop it into the oven until the cheese melts. Two halves contain 210 calories.

Junk Food

360 CALORIES

BBQ CHICKEN PIZZA

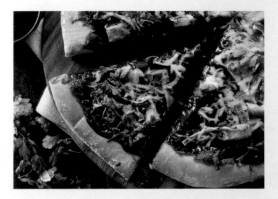

If you have a love affair with barbecue chicken pizza (you know who you are), it might break your heart to learn that a single small slice at some of the popular chains will cost you 360 calories. Do some quick math: that's 720 calories for two slices, and 1,080 for three . . . kind of hard to swallow.

Take a break from the pizza-chain version and give my low-carb recipe a try. The payoff? A downward trend in the numbers when it comes to your blood sugars and the bathroom scale.

Joy Food

240 CALORIES

BBQ CHICKEN PIZZA

makes 1 serving

By losing the doughy crust and replacing it with thinly pounded chicken marinated in barbecue sauce, you can enjoy an entire personal pie with the same delicious flavor for a fraction of the carbs. You also benefit from a hearty dose of energizing protein. Don't forget to pile on your favorite veggies to boost the fiber and antioxidants.

> One 5-ounce boneless, skinless chicken breast or cutlet
> ¼ cup barbecue sauce (any brand with no more than 40 calories per 2 tablespoons)
> ¼ bell pepper, thinly sliced
> ¼ onion, thinly sliced
> 2 tablespoons shredded part-skim mozzarella cheese

Pound the chicken breast very thin and marinate it in 2 tablespoons of the barbecue sauce for a couple of hours or overnight in the fridge. (To save time, you can buy thin-cut chicken breast.)

Preheat the oven to 375°F. Line a baking sheet with aluminum foil and coat the foil with nonstick oil spray.

Place the chicken on the baking sheet and put it in the oven for 15 minutes, or until fully cooked.

While the chicken is baking, coat a skillet with nonstick oil spray and sauté the bell pepper and onion over medium-high heat for about 7 minutes.

Top the cooked chicken with 2 tablespoons barbecue sauce, sautéed vegetables, cheese, and preferred seasonings. Place the chicken back in the oven until the cheese is melted and bubbly, about 3 minutes.

---

nutrition information PER SERVING
240 calories ▪ 34 g protein ▪ 5.5 g total fat (3.5 g unsaturated, 2 g saturated) ▪ 111 mg cholesterol ▪ 12.5 g carbs ▪ 2.5 g fiber
7.5 g total sugar (3.5 g natural, 4 g added) ▪ 650 mg sodium

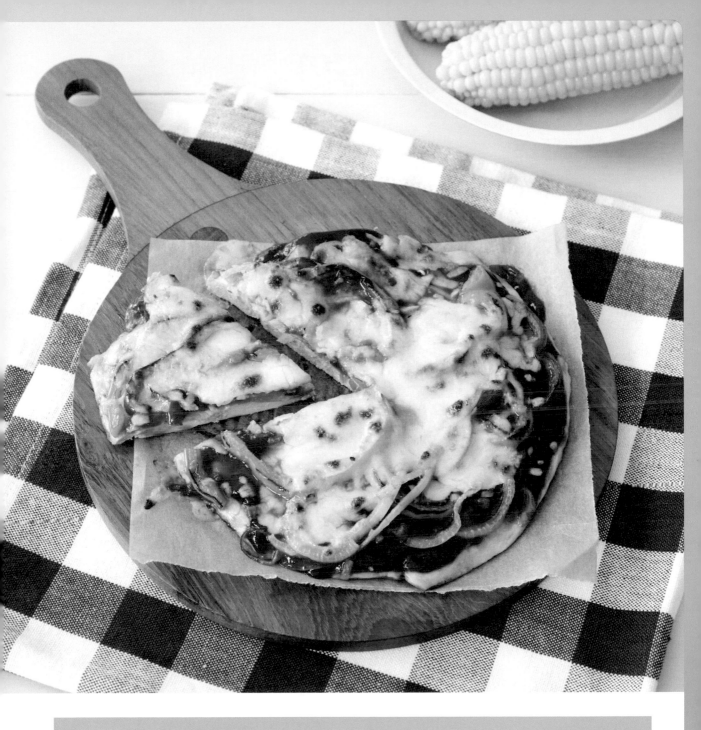

TASTY TWIST Elevate the barbecue experience with these unique serving suggestions. Before placing your chicken pizza in the oven, add 2 tablespoons of each: corn and my Seasoned Black Beans (page 135) evenly over the top. Or add a few tablespoons of my Better Baked Beans (page 90) and serve with my Coleslaw (page 108) on the side.

Junk Food

1,150 CALORIES

SPAGHETTI AND MEATBALLS

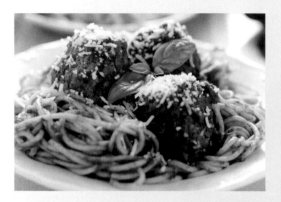

Nothing says comfort like a big bowl of noodles topped with meatballs, garlicky tomato sauce, and fresh grated cheese. However, a serving of spaghetti and meatballs at a restaurant is typically enough to feed two people—or, in some supersized instances, a small family. If you eat it all in one sitting, you'll be gobbling down 1,150 calories and about an entire day's worth of sodium.

I gave this pasta dish a friendly health makeover, so you can enjoy the same flavor minus the guilt. It's waaaay slimmer than the original—if it were a person, I'd guesstimate it dropped about 10 pant sizes!

Joy Food

411 CALORIES

ZUCCHINI LINGUINE WITH MEATBALLS

makes 4 servings

Using zucchini "noodles" instead of traditional pasta helps drive down calories and carbs while simultaneously beefing up the fiber and nutrients. Preparing flavorful meatballs with lean ground turkey and heart-healthy oats makes this dish a surprisingly guilt-free comfort food. Bonus: Because this recipe makes a nice big batch of meatballs, you'll have plenty left over for future lunches and dinners. You make 34 meatballs, but use only 16!

TURKEY MEATBALLS
1 medium onion, finely chopped
1 medium carrot, peeled and finely chopped
    or grated
2 cloves garlic, minced, or ½ teaspoon garlic powder
¾ cup grated Parmesan cheese
1 tablespoon dried Italian herb blend or
    2 teaspoons dried basil plus 2 teaspoons
    dried oregano
¾ teaspoon kosher salt or coarse sea salt
¼ teaspoon ground black pepper
¼ teaspoon red pepper flakes
1¼ pounds ground turkey
    (at least 90 percent lean)
1 egg, lightly beaten
¼ cup old-fashioned or quick-cooking rolled oats
One 24-ounce jar marinara sauce, store-bought
    or homemade

ZUCCHINI LINGUINE
8 large zucchini
½ teaspoon garlic powder
Onion powder to taste
Salt and pepper to taste

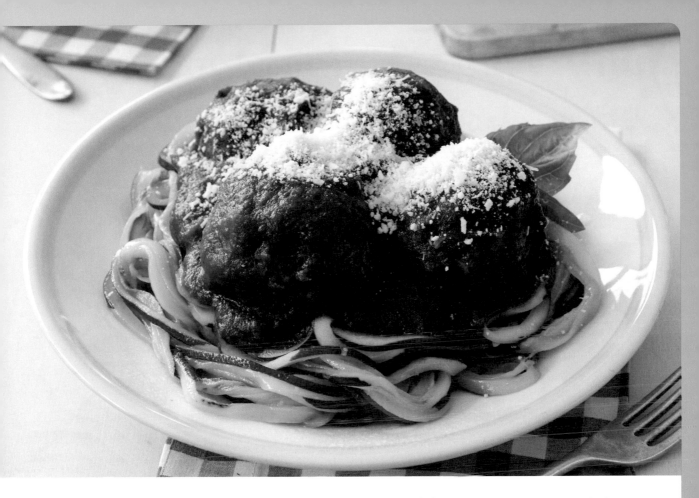

To make the meatballs, combine the onion, carrot, garlic, Parmesan cheese, Italian herb blend, salt, pepper, and red pepper flakes in a large mixing bowl.

Add the ground turkey, egg, and oats. Mix until the ingredients are well combined.

Shape the meat mixture into about 34 meatballs, about 1½ inches in diameter, and carefully place them one at a time into a large pot with the marinara sauce. Do not stir; stirring will cause the meatballs to break apart. Do not worry if some of the meatballs are not completely submerged in the sauce. Cover the pot and simmer on medium-low heat for 20 minutes.

Remove the lid and gently stir the meatballs to thoroughly coat them with the sauce. Continue to simmer, uncovered, for an additional 20 minutes.

To make the zucchini linguine, while the meatballs are cooking, cut off the ends of the zucchini and julienne using a spiral slicer to create noodle strands. (You can peel the zucchini or leave the skin intact.) If you don't have a spiral slicer, use a vegetable peeler or knife. Wrap noodle strands in a few layers of paper towels and squeeze to remove some of the moisture.

Liberally coat a large skillet with nonstick oil spray and warm over medium heat. Add the zucchini linguine, garlic powder, and onion powder, and sauté for 2 minutes. Season with salt and pepper. Drain the liquid and divide among 4 plates. Top each plate with 4 meatballs and the sauce.

nutrition information PER SERVING OF 2 CUPS LINGUINE AND 4 MEATBALLS ▪ 411 calories ▪ 49 g protein ▪ 10.5 g total fat (6 g unsaturated, 4.5 g saturated) ▪ 140 mg cholesterol ▪ 31 g carbs ▪ 7 g fiber ▪ 17 g total sugar (17 g natural, 0 g added) ▪ 900 mg sodium

Junk Food

750 CALORIES

VEGGIE LASAGNA

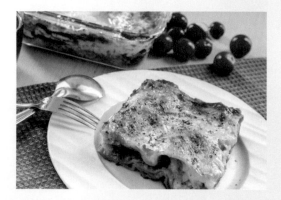

Think you're safe with a nice slice of vegetable lasagna? Not so fast. A generous helping can pack as many as 750 calories. Sure, there are some veggies in there, but you'll probably have to look under gobs of full-fat cheese and layers of starchy noodles to find them.

Good news for meat-free lasagna lovers: I've dramatically lightened up this comfort-food favorite with a few simple tricks here and there. Plus, I've packed in lots of fiber-rich spinach and pulled back on the starch. And thanks to a clever strategy that I learned from my mom, there's no need to precook the noodles, which makes dinner prep a snap.

Joy Food

220 CALORIES

SPINACH LASAGNA

makes 12 servings

My ooey-gooey, cheesy Spinach Lasagna will hit the spot. It's slim and scrumptious, and it's perfect for a simple weeknight supper or for serving company. Thanks to the heaps of frozen spinach, there's a whole lot of nutrients and fiber In every luscious bite.

> Two 10-ounce boxes frozen, chopped spinach
> 2 cups part-skim ricotta cheese
> 1 egg
> 1 egg white
> ½ teaspoon ground black pepper
> 1 teaspoon garlic powder or 4 cloves garlic, minced
> ½ teaspoon dried basil
> ½ teaspoon dried oregano
> One 24-ounce jar tomato sauce or marinara sauce, store-bought or homemade
> 9 whole-grain lasagna noodles, uncooked
> 2 cups shredded part-skim mozzarella cheese

Preheat the oven to 350°F. Coat a 9 x 13–inch baking dish with nonstick oil spray.

Cook the spinach according to package directions and squeeze out the water. Set aside.

In a large bowl, mix together the ricotta cheese, egg, egg white, pepper, garlic powder, basil, and oregano. Add the spinach and mix again thoroughly.

Cover the bottom of the pan with tomato sauce (about one-quarter of the jar) and place down 3 of the uncooked lasagna noodles. Top with half of the spinach-ricotta mixture and then a layer of 3 more noodles. Top with the remaining spinach-ricotta mixture and then the remaining 3 lasagna noodles. Pour the remaining tomato sauce on top.

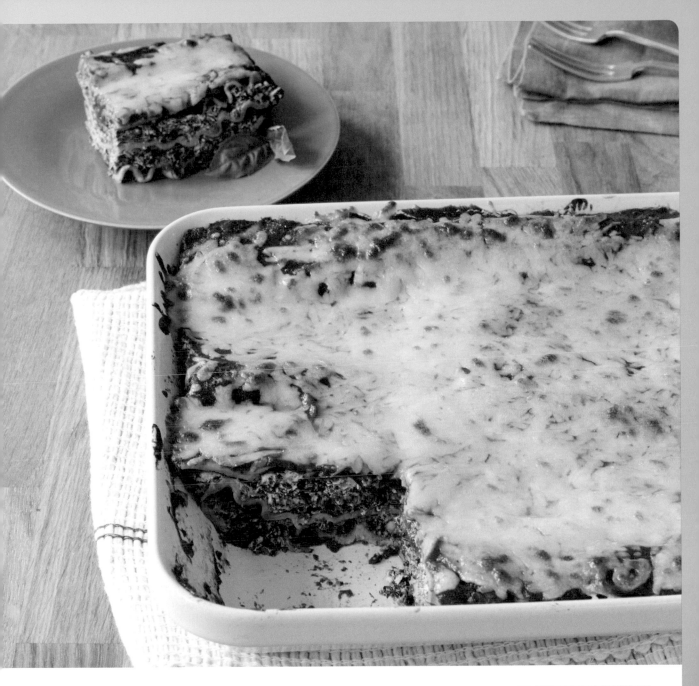

Sprinkle on the mozzarella cheese. Pour about ½ cup of water around the edge of the pan (this will cook the noodles), and cover the pan tightly with aluminum foil.

Bake for 45 minutes. Remove the foil and bake uncovered for 30 more minutes. Let cool for 10 to 15 minutes before slicing to allow the lasagna to set and the extra water to be absorbed.

nutrition information PER SERVING
220 calories ▪ 15 g protein ▪ 8 g total fat (4 g unsaturated, 4 g saturated) ▪ 38 mg cholesterol ▪ 22 g carbs ▪ 5 g fiber 4 g total sugar (4 g natural, 0 g added) ▪ 370 mg sodium

Junk Food

1,310 CALORIES

MAC AND CHEESE

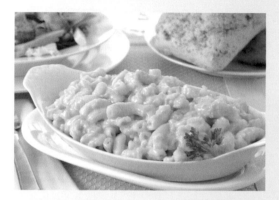

You'd be hard-pressed to find somebody who doesn't love a good old-fashioned bowl of mac and cheese. But sadly, this drool-worthy comfort food is loaded with gobs of butter, heavy cream, and full-fat cheese. Order it at a restaurant and you'll be spooning up a whopping 1,310 calories.

You can make this dish light 'n' lean by cooking it at home. My recipe is quick, easy, and definitely kid approved (Bauer-kid approved, neighborhood-kid approved—even finicky-foodie approved). Feel free to add some steamed broccoli florets or cooked carrots to the mix for an extra kick of nutrients and fiber.

Joy Food

419 CALORIES

MAC AND CHEESE
makes 6 servings

This recipe has earned rock-star status at countless dinner parties and family get-togethers. I owe all the credit to my youngest daughter, Ayden Jane, who would not sign off on a final version until it met her "OMG, this is amazing" seal of approval. The end result is an incredibly delectable, melted-cheesy macaroni dish that will most definitely hit the spot.

> One 14-ounce box whole-grain elbow macaroni
> 2¼ cups skim milk
> 1 teaspoon reduced-sodium soy sauce
> 1 teaspoon onion powder
> ½ teaspoon dry mustard
> ¼ teaspoon paprika
> 1 bay leaf
> ½ teaspoon kosher salt or coarse sea salt
> ⅛ teaspoon ground black pepper
> 3 to 5 drops hot sauce
> 1 tablespoon cornstarch
> 10 ounces (or 2½ cups) shredded reduced-fat sharp cheddar cheese
> 2 tablespoons whipped butter or trans-fat-free buttery spread

Bring a large pot of water to a boil. Add the macaroni and follow the directions on the package for al dente pasta.

While the macaroni is cooking, prepare the cheese sauce: In a large saucepan, combine 2 cups of the milk with the soy sauce, onion powder, dry mustard, paprika, bay leaf, salt, pepper, and hot sauce. Place the mixture over medium heat, and cook until it comes to a gentle simmer.

In a small bowl or cup, mix the cornstarch with the remaining ¼ cup milk. Add the cornstarch mixture to

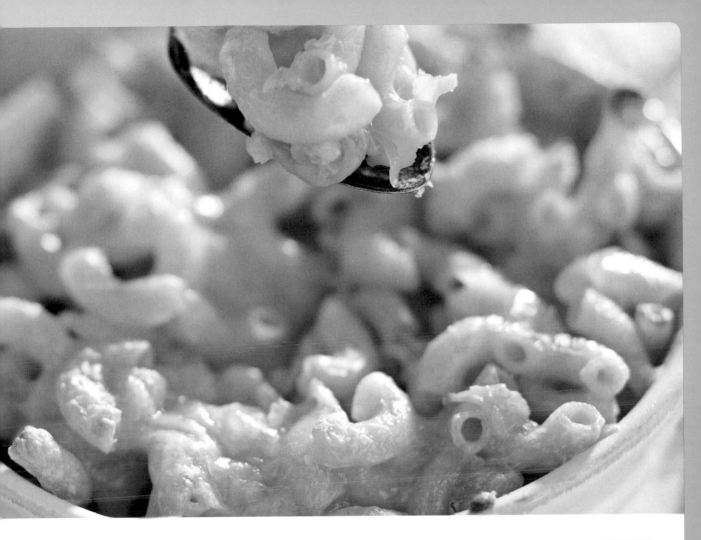

the saucepan and stir to combine. Return the sauce to a simmer and cook for 2 to 3 minutes, stirring occasionally, until slightly thick.

Remove the saucepan from the heat, discard the bay leaf, and add the shredded cheese. Stir until the cheese is completely melted and no lumps remain.

Add the butter to the cheese sauce and stir until it is completely melted and combined.

Drain the macaroni (do not rinse), and return it to the pot.

Pour the cheese sauce over the cooked macaroni and stir until everything is coated. Cover the pot with a tight-fitting lid and let the macaroni and cheese to sit for 10 minutes, to allow the sauce to thicken before serving.

nutrition information PER 1½-CUP SERVING
419 calories ▪ 25 g protein ▪ 13 g total fat (7 g unsaturated, 6 g saturated) ▪ 35 mg cholesterol ▪ 58 g carbs ▪ 6 g fiber 4.5 g total sugar (4.5 g natural, 0 g added) ▪ 680 mg sodium

TASTY TWIST For baked macaroni and cheese with a crispy, crunchy top: After combining the cheese sauce with the cooked macaroni, transfer the mac and cheese to a 9 x 13-inch baking dish coated with nonstick oil spray. Sprinkle ¼ cup of grated Parmesan cheese evenly over the top. Place the pan under a preheated broiler for 4 to 7 minutes, or until the top is golden brown and crispy; check often to make sure the cheese does not burn.

Junk Food

PESTO PASTA

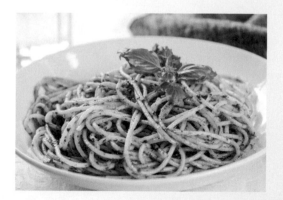

Although pesto sauce is composed of healthy ingredients, a few of its signature items are super calorie-dense (ahem, olive oil, pine nuts, Parm). And when mixed with a mound of starchy noodles, pesto pasta becomes pasta-trocious. One big bowl can easily top 1,220 calories.

I've been hard at work trying to turn this cherished entrée into a diet-friendly dish. Happy news for pesto enthusiasts: With a few simple substitutions, you can still enjoy my recipe without breaking the calorie bank. Mission accomplished.

Joy Food

ZUCCHINI LINGUINE WITH PESTO

makes 4 servings

By swapping spaghetti for julienned zucchini and replacing oil with vegetable broth, I've transformed this dish into a health-enhancing entrée. While it's significantly lighter in calories, carbs, fat, and salt, this new and improved version is still fabulous, filling, and flavorful. And of course, the sauce works beautifully tossed with traditional pasta as well.

PESTO SAUCE
4 cups loosely packed fresh basil
¼ cup grated Parmesan cheese
3 cloves garlic, quartered
½ cup reduced-sodium vegetable or chicken broth
1 teaspoon kosher salt or coarse sea salt
¼ teaspoon ground black pepper

ZUCCHINI LINGUINE
8 large zucchini
½ teaspoon garlic powder
Onion powder to taste
Salt and pepper to taste

TOPPINGS
½ cup Parmesan cheese
Halved cherry tomatoes (optional)

To make the pesto sauce, combine the basil, Parmesan cheese, garlic, broth, salt, and pepper in a food processor or blender and mix to form a loose paste. Set the pesto sauce aside.

To make the zucchini linguine, cut off the ends of the zucchini and julienne using a spiral slicer to create noodle strands. If you don't have a spiral slicer, use a vegetable peeler or knife. (You can peel the zucchini

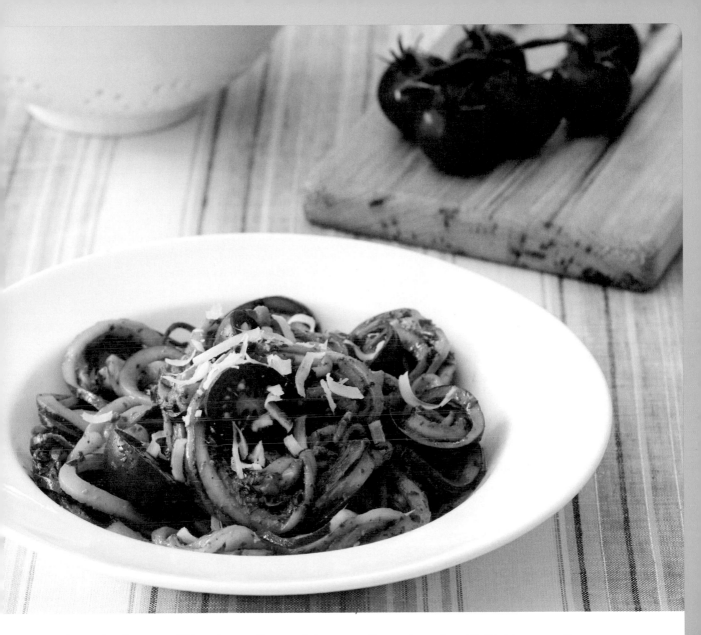

or leave the skin intact.) Wrap the noodle strands in a few layers of paper towels and squeeze to remove some of the moisture.

In a large skillet coated with nonstick oil spray, sauté the zucchini linguine over medium heat with the garlic and onion powder for about 2 minutes. Add the pesto sauce and stir to combine. Season with salt and pepper to taste.

Top each serving with 2 tablespoons Parmesan cheese, or simply toss it directly into the pasta and mix thoroughly before serving.

Pour the halved cherry tomatoes over the pasta for a pretty pop of color, if desired, and serve.

nutrition information PER 2-CUP SERVING
135 calories ▪ 11 g protein ▪ 5 g total fat (2 g unsaturated, 3 g saturated) ▪ 17 mg cholesterol ▪ 10 g carbs ▪ 4 g fiber 6.5 g total sugar (6.5 g natural, 0 g added) ▪ 610 mg sodium

Junk Food

1,090 CALORIES

FETTUCCINE ALFREDO

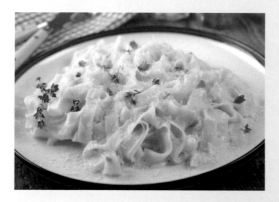

Pasta doused in heavy cream, Parmesan cheese, and butter is a diet disaster. One heaping bowl of indulgent fettuccine Alfredo at your favorite Italian restaurant can tally up to more than 1,000 calories and 41 grams of saturated fat. (You may want to keep your cardiologist on speed dial—that's the saturated fat equivalent of ¾ of a stick of butter.)

My lighter take on the classic is just as rich and delicious, but for half the calories (yes, for real). Go ahead and give it a try.

Joy Food

364 CALORIES

FETTUCCINE ALFREDO

makes 5 servings

If you're in the mood for decadent, cheesy, and incredibly creamy pasta, you're on the right page. It takes just four simple ingredients to transform fettuccine Alfredo from fat to fit—no fancy footwork required. Couple a hearty 2-cup serving with a tossed salad and buckle in for an amazing meal.

> One 12-ounce box whole-grain linguine or fettuccine
> One 12-ounce can fat-free evaporated milk
> 3 ounces (6 tablespoons) light or reduced-fat cream cheese, at room temperature
> ½ teaspoon kosher salt or coarse sea salt
> ¼ teaspoon ground black pepper
> ½ cup grated Parmesan cheese

Bring a large pot of water to a boil. Cook the pasta according to the package instructions.

While the pasta cooks, prepare the Alfredo sauce: In a 2-quart saucepan, combine the evaporated milk, cream cheese, salt, and pepper. Place the saucepan over medium-low heat and cook, stirring occasionally with a wire whisk to break up the cream cheese, until the cream cheese is completely melted and the mixture is barely simmering, 5 to 7 minutes. Be careful not to overheat the mixture because the milk will curdle.

Stir in the Parmesan cheese and whisk for 1 minute. Remove the Alfredo sauce from the heat.

Drain the pasta, reserving approximately 1 cup of the cooking water.

Add the pasta back to the pot, pour on the Alfredo sauce, and toss to coat. Season with extra salt and plenty of pepper. Serve immediately.

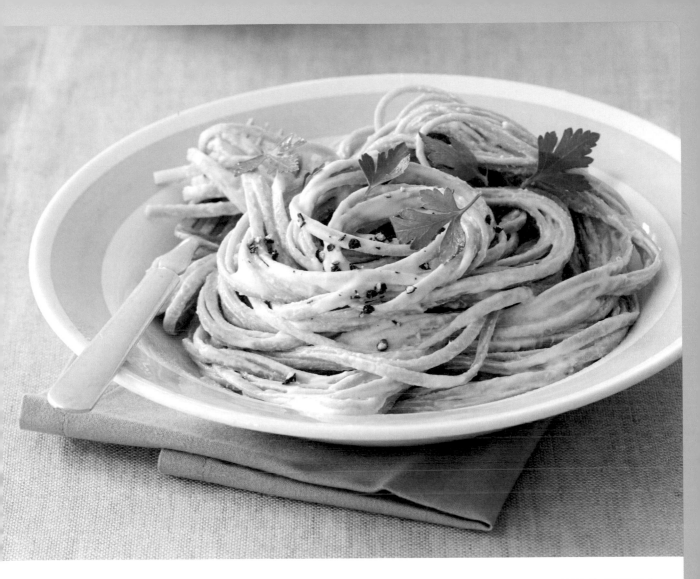

If you are not able to serve right away, the sauce will begin to thicken as it stands. Simply thin it out with the reserved pasta water, adding it in ¼-cup increments until the desired consistency is achieved.

Note: Because the sauce thickens in the fridge, I recommend adding a splash of water or milk when reheating leftovers. Microwave and stir before serving.

nutrition information PER 2-CUP SERVING
364 calories ▪ 20 g protein ▪ 6.5 g total fat (3 g unsaturated, 3.5 g saturated) ▪ 20 mg cholesterol ▪ 52 g carbs ▪ 7 g fiber 9 g total sugar (9 g natural, 0 g added) ▪ 452 mg sodium

SERVE IT UP SLIM **Use squash instead of noodles! Microwave a spaghetti squash for 4 minutes to soften. Slice off ends; then slice in half lengthwise. Scoop out seeds and pulp. Place squash (cut side down) in a baking dish with an inch of water. Microwave for 10 minutes. Once cool, use a fork to scrape out spaghetti-like strands and toss with a little Alfredo sauce. Or forego the Alfredo and sauté the "spaghetti" in a skillet coated with nonstick oil spray. Season with salt, pepper, garlic, onion powder, and a few tablespoons of marinara sauce and Parm (60 calories per cup).**

Junk Food

COLD SESAME NOODLES

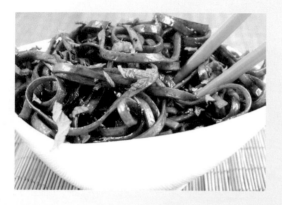

These noodles may be served chilled, but they are definitely not the light and refreshing dish you're looking for on a hot summer day. Combine starchy pasta, sesame oil, and peanut butter, and you have yourself a not-so-cool 780 calories per order.

My healthy spin is a mainstay in the Bauer house because my kids—and their friends—are constantly requesting it. It packs the same peanut-butter punch without the blow to your waistline.

Joy Food

COLD SESAME NOODLES

makes 4 servings

Skip the Chinese takeout. This slimmed-down spaghetti is filled with oodles of sesame and peanut-buttery goodness. Thanks to a little recipe makeover magic, you can now enjoy this dish's authentic flavor without the guilt. Eat it hot or cold, with or without the veggies—it's delicious and nutritious either way.

> One 12-ounce box whole-grain spaghetti
> 2 teaspoons toasted sesame oil
> 3 tablespoons natural peanut butter
> ¼ cup low-sodium chicken or vegetable broth
> ¼ cup reduced-sodium soy sauce
> 1 tablespoon sugar
> 1 tablespoon rice wine vinegar
> ½ teaspoon hot sauce (optional)
> 1 small cucumber, peeled, seeded, and diced (optional)
> 6 baby carrots, chopped (optional)
> 3 scallions (green onions), thinly sliced (optional)
> Ground black pepper to taste

Bring a large pot of water to a boil. Cook the spaghetti until al dente according to package directions. Drain the spaghetti, transfer it to a large mixing bowl, and toss the noodles with the sesame oil.

In a small bowl, whisk together the peanut butter, broth, soy sauce, sugar, vinegar, and hot sauce, if desired, until smooth.

Pour the peanut-butter sauce over the noodles and toss well, making sure the noodles thoroughly soak up all the sauce on the bottom of the bowl. Add the cucumber, carrots, and half of the scallions, if

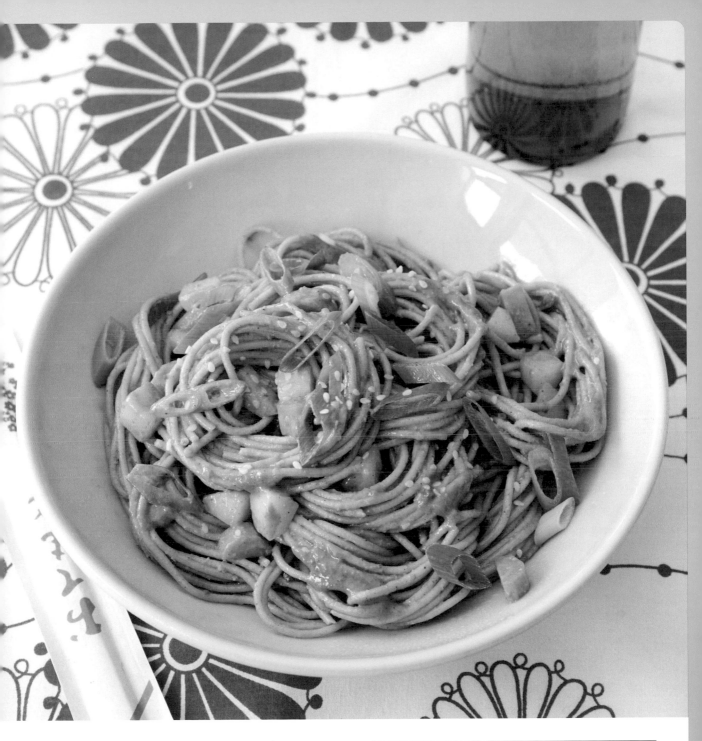

desired. Toss to combine and season with pepper. Spoon the noodles into a serving bowl and top with the remaining scallions, if desired. Serve hot, cold, or at room temperature.

nutrition information PER 1½-CUP SERVING
407 calories ▪ 16 g protein ▪ 9.5 g total fat (8 g unsaturated, 1.5 g saturated) ▪ 0 mg cholesterol ▪ 71 g carbs ▪ 9 g fiber 4 g total sugar (1 g natural, 3 g added) ▪ 350 mg sodium

Junk Food

VEGETABLE LO MEIN

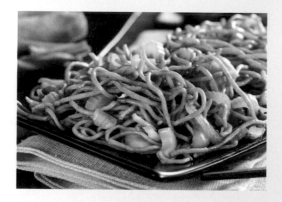

Ordering Chinese? You may think vegetable lo mein is a diet-friendly dish because, hey, *vegetable* is right there in the title. But there are many more noodles than veggies, and the dish is usually made with a lot of oil. A cup of lo mein can cost you about 325 calories—and who stops at 1 cup?! Admittedly, not me.

I decided to make a low-carb, yummy version using zucchini noodles. I added in a bunch of other veggies and created a dish with a lot of volume and fiber for a fraction of the calorie cost.

Joy Food

90 CALORIES

VEGETABLE LO MEIN

makes 4 servings

Drop the take-out menu! Whip up this delicious Vegetable Lo Mein with zucchini noodles to cut the carbs and calories without cutting the flavor. Serve it as a side dish or toss in some diced chicken, beef, seafood, or baked tofu for a healthy (and tasty) meal.

   4 large zucchini
   1 onion, sliced
   3 cloves garlic, minced, or ¾ teaspoon
      garlic powder
   1 tablespoon grated fresh ginger,
      or ¾ teaspoon ground ginger
   1 red, yellow, or orange bell pepper, sliced
   1 medium carrot, shredded
   2 teaspoons toasted sesame oil
   4 tablespoons reduced-sodium soy sauce
   Ground black pepper to taste
   Hot sauce (optional)
   1 scallion (green onion), sliced, for garnish

To make zucchini noodles, cut off the ends of the zucchini and julienne using a spiral slicer to create noodle strands. If you don't have a spiral slicer, use a vegetable peeler or knife. (You can peel the zucchini or leave the skin intact.) Wrap the noodle strands in a few layers of paper towels and squeeze to remove some of the moisture.

Liberally coat a large skillet with nonstick oil spray and warm it over medium heat. Sauté the onion, stirring frequently, until it is slightly browned.

Add the garlic, ginger, and bell pepper. Continue to cook, stirring occasionally, for about 5 minutes, or until the pepper is tender. Add the carrot, sesame oil, and 2 tablespoons of the soy sauce. Continue to cook for an additional 3 minutes.

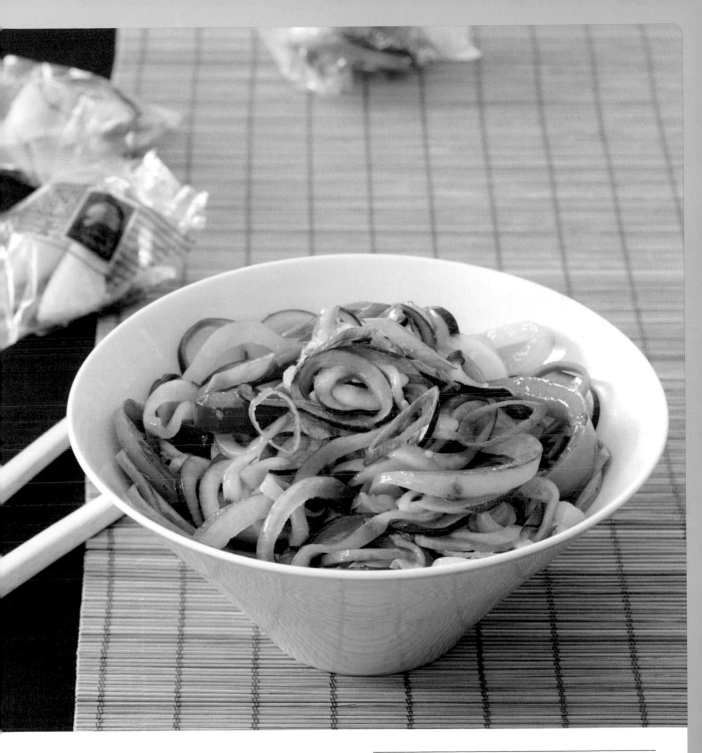

Finally, add in the zucchini and the remaining 2 tablespoons soy sauce. Cook for about 2 minutes, or until zucchini noodles are tender. Add pepper and hot sauce, if desired. Serve with scallions on top.

nutrition information PER 1-CUP SERVING
90 calories ▪ 5 g protein ▪ 3 g total fat (2.5 g unsaturated, 0.5 g saturated) ▪ 0 mg cholesterol ▪ 13 g carbs ▪ 3.5 g fiber 8 g total sugar (8 g natural, 0 g added) ▪ 460 mg sodium

Junk Food

CHEESY MEAT LASAGNA

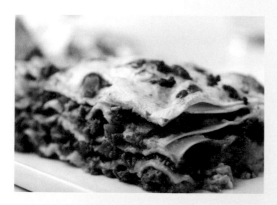

Classic lasagna marries two indulgent ingredients—meat and cheese (yum)—to create a crave-worthy and crowd-pleasing meal. Unfortunately, this decadent dish is typically oozing with calories, approximately 960 per hearty helping. Holy lasagna!

Instead, you can dig in and stay healthy with my trim take, which features the same yummy flavors without any of the bloating, heartburn, or regret.

Joy Food

235 CALORIES

CHEESY MEAT LASAGNA ROLLS

makes 14 servings

This recipe puts a creative spin on lasagna—it works just as well for a family supper as it does for a dinner party with guests. The great part about this indulgent dish is that it comes perfectly packaged—automatic portion control. And it freezes beautifully, so you can cook once and enjoy twice.

Don't be intimidated by the assembly. If you can make lasagna, you can make these rolls. And recruiting young sous chefs in the prep will make it all the more fun.

- 1½ cups fat-free or part-skim ricotta cheese
- 1½ cups shredded part-skim mozzarella cheese
- 1 egg, lightly beaten
- 1 teaspoon garlic powder
- 2 teaspoons dried oregano
- ½ teaspoon ground black pepper
- 1 pound lean ground turkey (at least 90 percent lean)
- One 24-ounce jar marinara sauce, store-bought or homemade
- 14 lasagna noodles, cooked al dente (7 to 8 minutes)
- ¼ cup grated Parmesan cheese
- ¼ teaspoon red pepper flakes (optional)

Preheat the oven to 425°F.

In a mixing bowl, combine the ricotta, ½ cup of the mozzarella, the egg, ¼ teaspoon of the garlic powder, the oregano, and the black pepper. Set aside.

In a large skillet coated with nonstick oil spray, cook the turkey meat over medium-high heat for about 8 minutes, stirring continually to break apart and crumble. Drain off the fat and discard.

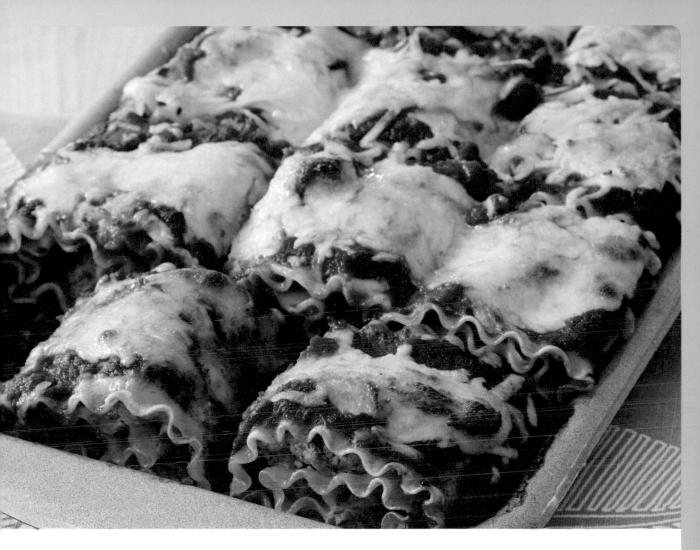

Stir in 1½ cups of the marinara sauce along with the remaining ¾ teaspoon of garlic powder. Mix thoroughly and remove from the heat.

Add the meat sauce to the cheese mixture and combine.

To assemble the lasagna rolls, cover the bottom of a casserole pan with a thin layer (about ½ cup) of marinara sauce.

On a flat work surface, lay out each noodle one at a time and add ¼ cup of the meat filling on top. Using your fingers, spread the filling evenly to cover the entire length of the noodle. Roll the noodle starting with the end closest to you. Place into the prepared casserole pan with the seam underneath so the lasagna noodles do not come unrolled.

When all of the noodles are neatly rolled and set in the pan, pour the remaining cup of the marinara sauce evenly over the top. Sprinkle with the remaining 1 cup mozzarella and top it with the grated Parmesan cheese and red pepper flakes, if desired.

Cover with foil and bake for 15 minutes. Uncover and bake for an additional 5 to 10 minutes, until the cheese is golden brown and bubbly.

nutrition information PER SERVING
235 calories ▪ 20 g protein ▪ 7 g total fat (4 g unsaturated, 3 g saturated) ▪ 47 mg cholesterol ▪ 23 g carbs ▪ 4.5 g fiber 3 g total sugar (3 g natural, 0 g added) ▪ 300 mg sodium

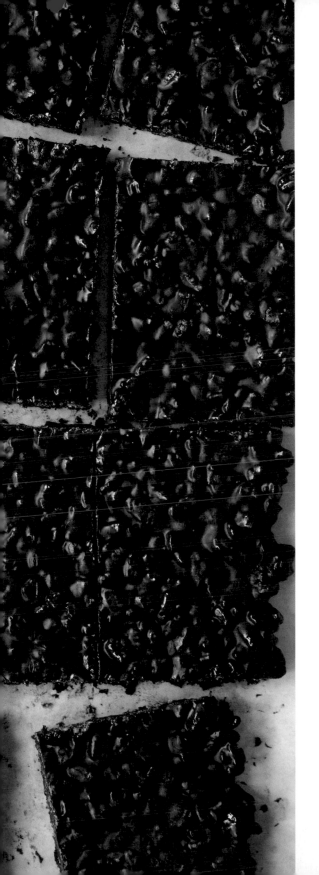

Chapter 7

DECADENT DESSERTS

Death by chocolate . . . or vanilla . . . or mint chocolate chip . . . or apple pie . . . or cheesecake. Pick your poison, because really, no matter which indulgence you choose, you're in for it, right?

Happily, no! You can savor all your favorite sweets—from cakes and pies to cupcakes and brownies—and still keep it slim with the diet-friendly desserts that fill the coming pages. Enjoy a tasty twist on key lime pie, slurp down a chocolate milkshake without going into calorie overload, and satisfy your sweet tooth with indulgent peanut butter cups made from wholesome ingredients.

As a lover of sweets myself, I spent a lot of time on this particular part of the cookbook. It's my favorite section, which means it's the longest. You're welcome.

Junk Food

450 CALORIES

PEACH MELBA

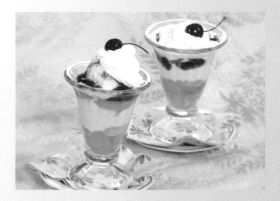

When a dessert features fruit, it can't be that bad . . . right? Wrong. Consider the traditional peach melba. The sugar, ice cream, and raspberry syrup incorporated in this dish make it a calorie catastrophe, with 450 per serving.

But you can whip up my three-ingredient Peach Melba makeover any day of the week. It has only 90 calories and all the sweet flavor of the original.

Joy Food

90 CALORIES

PEACH MELBA

makes 2 servings

This dish was a cinch to slim down: Peaches are naturally sweet, and you can bring out that sweetness even more by throwing them on the grill, so there's no need to add extra sugar. Replace the caloric ice cream with creamy Greek yogurt (or vanilla frozen yogurt) and the raspberry sauce with fresh raspberries, and the result is great taste and *big* savings.

This quick recipe works as an easy treat to serve the family after dinner, and it doubles as an elegant dessert for guests at a get-together. And all for just 90 calories!

> 1 ripe peach
> ½ cup nonfat vanilla Greek yogurt or vanilla frozen yogurt
> ½ cup fresh or frozen raspberries

Spray the grill or grill pan with nonstick oil spray and warm to medium-high heat.

Slice the peach in half and remove the pit. Place the cut sides down on the grill and allow to cook until the peaches start to caramelize, but are still firm, 2 to 3 minutes.

Remove the peaches from the heat, add a dollop of yogurt to each half, and top with raspberries.

---

nutrition information PER SERVING
90 calories ▪ 7 g protein ▪ 0 g total fat (0 g unsaturated, 0 g saturated) ▪ 0 mg cholesterol ▪ 16.5 g carbs ▪ 3.5 g fiber 13 g total sugar (9.5 g natural, 3.5 g added) ▪ 25 mg sodium

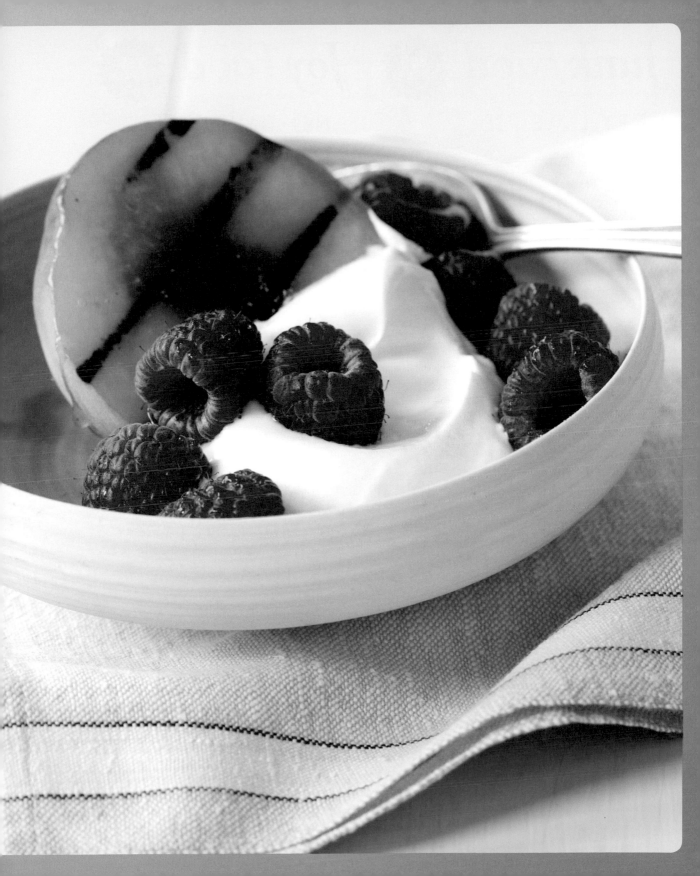

Junk Food

KEY LIME PIE

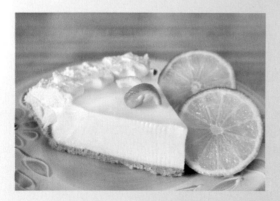

Key lime pie might seem like a lighter choice at the dessert table compared with cheesecake or death by chocolate, but don't be fooled. A slice can pack as many as 500 calories—with some versions as high as 690!

Sure, you can control the ingredients and nutrition when you bake at home, but who has the time to prep the crust, whip up the filling, and then make the whipped cream topping?

My No-Bake Key Lime Pie gives you the same citrus flavor of the decadent dessert for far fewer calories and significantly less effort—you don't even have to turn on the oven. Nice deal, right?

Joy Food

NO-BAKE KEY LIME PIE

makes 1 serving

What's not to love about this dessert? It's full of flavor, low in calories, and packed with protein. It's also a snap to make. Grab a spoon and dig in.

> One 5- to 6-ounce container nonfat plain Greek yogurt
> Juice of 4 key limes or 1 regular lime
> 1½ teaspoons sugar
> 1 graham cracker square, crushed
> 1 slice lime (optional)

Mix the yogurt, key lime juice, and sugar in a small bowl.

Sprinkle the crushed graham cracker crumbs on top.

Garnished with the slice of lime, if desired.

---

nutrition information PER SERVING
165 calories ▪ 18 g protein ▪ 1 g total fat (1 g unsaturated, 0 g saturated) ▪ 10 mg cholesterol ▪ 21 g carbs ▪ 0.5 g fiber 14 g total sugar (8 g natural, 6 g added) ▪ 90 mg sodium

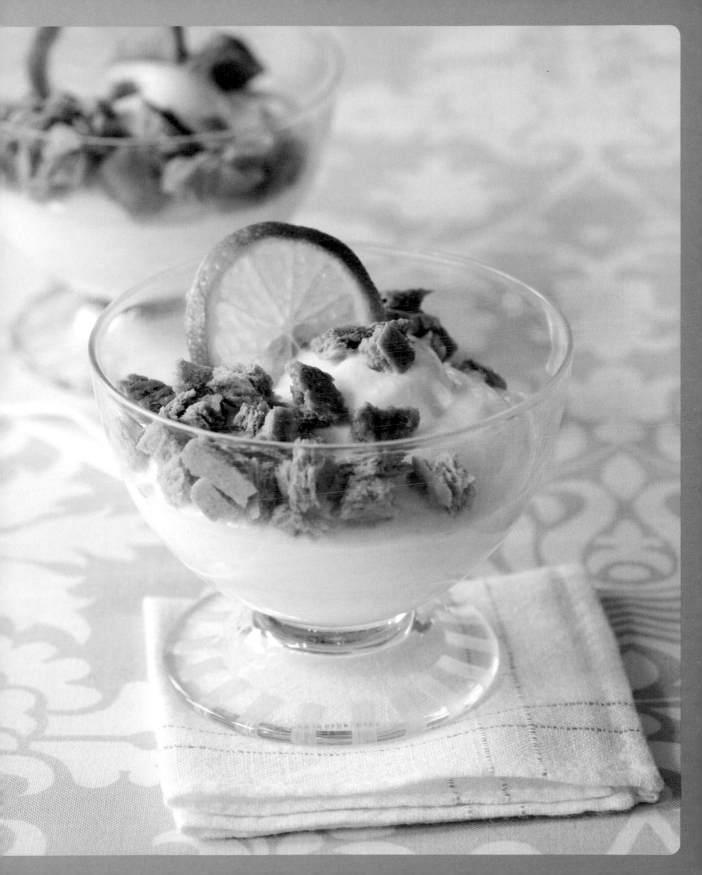

Junk Food

CREAM-FILLED CHOCOLATE CAKES

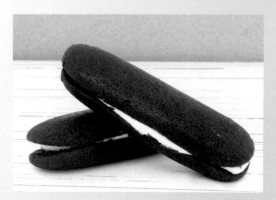

You may recognize this treat as the childhood classic with the devilish name. Each chocolate-whipped cream memory comes with a 180-calorie price tag, more than 4 teaspoons of added sugar, and a not-so-angelic ingredient list including high fructose corn syrup, refined flour, and partially hydrogenated oil, which is code for damaging trans fat.

But you can still enjoy a taste of the good old days with my better-for-you snack cakes, which taste . . . heavenly, of course.

Joy Food

140 CALORIES

CREAM-FILLED CHOCOLATE CAKES

makes 10 servings

On a mission to create a lightened-up version of this nostalgic treat, I sandwiched airy whipped cream between two irresistible chocolaty cakes made with wholesome ingredients (and some TLC). For just 140 calories, my homemade version delivers sweet satisfaction without any guilt. Word of caution: squirt the whipped cream and add the top half right before serving, or they'll flatten out.

1½ cups white whole-wheat flour or
    whole-wheat pastry flour
½ teaspoon kosher salt or coarse sea salt
1 teaspoon baking powder
1 teaspoon baking soda
6 tablespoons unsweetened cocoa powder
¾ cup unsweetened applesauce
¾ cup skim milk
½ cup sugar
3 egg whites
1 teaspoon vanilla extract
Canned whipped topping

Preheat the oven to 325°F. Prepare 4 standard loaf pans with nonstick oil spray.

In a large bowl, whisk together the flour, salt, baking powder, baking soda, and cocoa powder.

In a separate medium bowl, whisk together the applesauce, milk, sugar, egg whites, and vanilla.

Add the wet ingredients to the dry ingredients and fold the batter until just combined.

Pour a very small layer of batter evenly into each of the 4 prepared pans and bake for 15 to 18 minutes, or until a toothpick inserted into the center of the loaf comes out clean.

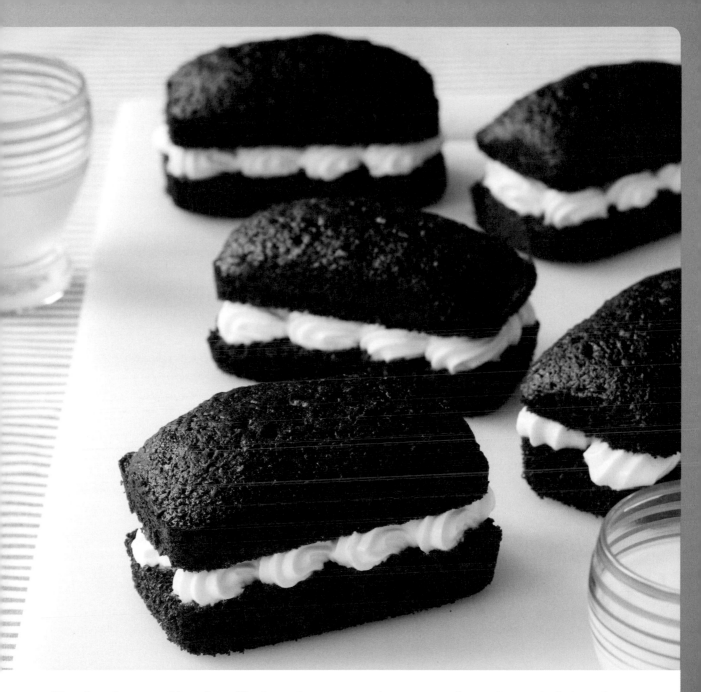

Allow the cakes to cool for at least 30 minutes in the pans. Cut each cake into 5 pieces, crosswise, creating mini chocolate cakes. Carefully remove each and place it on a platter or plate.

Squirt the whipped cream (about 2 tablespoons' worth) along the top of 1 chocolate cake strip and gently top with another. Repeat with the remaining cakes or save and store them in the fridge or freezer and enjoy at another time.

nutrition information PER SERVING
140 calories ▪ 5 g protein ▪ 2 g total fat (1 g unsaturated, 1 g saturated) ▪ 0 mg cholesterol ▪ 28 g carbs ▪ 2.5 g fiber 13.5 g total sugar (3 g natural, 10.5 g added) ▪ 290 mg sodium

Junk Food

600 CALORIES

BOSTON CREAM PIE

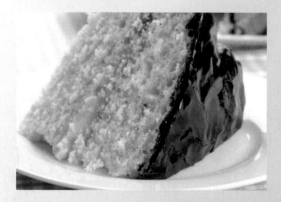

The traditional Boston cream pie, which was created at the Parker House Hotel in Boston (of course), consists of eggs, sugar, butter, milk, flour, and chocolate. A single standard slice clocks in at a whopping 600 calories—beating out many other dessert items on the menu.

If you're looking for the classic taste and are willing to downscale your portion, my parfait rendition is the way to go. It features all the same flavors but in a smaller and innovative presentation.

Joy Food

185 CALORIES

BOSTON CREAM PIE PARFAIT

makes 6 servings

This recipe transforms the calorie-laden Boston cream pie into a diet-friendly dessert. It layers a creamy vanilla pudding with crumbled graham crackers and a warm chocolate sauce. In the spirit of Boston, it's *wicked wonderful*.

PUDDING
⅓ cup sugar
3 tablespoons cornstarch or arrowroot flour
⅛ teaspoon salt
2 cups skim milk
2 egg yolks
1 tablespoon vanilla

TOPPING
¼ cup semisweet chocolate chips
6 graham cracker squares (3 long strips)

To make the pudding: Mix the sugar, cornstarch, and salt in a medium saucepan. Gradually stir in the milk until the cornstarch is completely dissolved. Cook over medium heat, stirring constantly, until the mixture thickens and boils, about 8 minutes.

In a small bowl, lightly beat the egg yolks. Slowly pour and mix about half of the hot milk mixture into the yolks, and then stir this mixture back into the hot saucepan with the rest of the milk mixture. Bring to a boil, stir for 1 minute, and remove the pan from the heat. Stir in the vanilla and divide the pudding among four ramekins. Refrigerate for at least 1 hour to chill and firm.

To assemble the parfaits: Remove the pudding from the fridge. Melt the chocolate chips in the microwave, stopping to stir every 15 to 30 seconds, until the

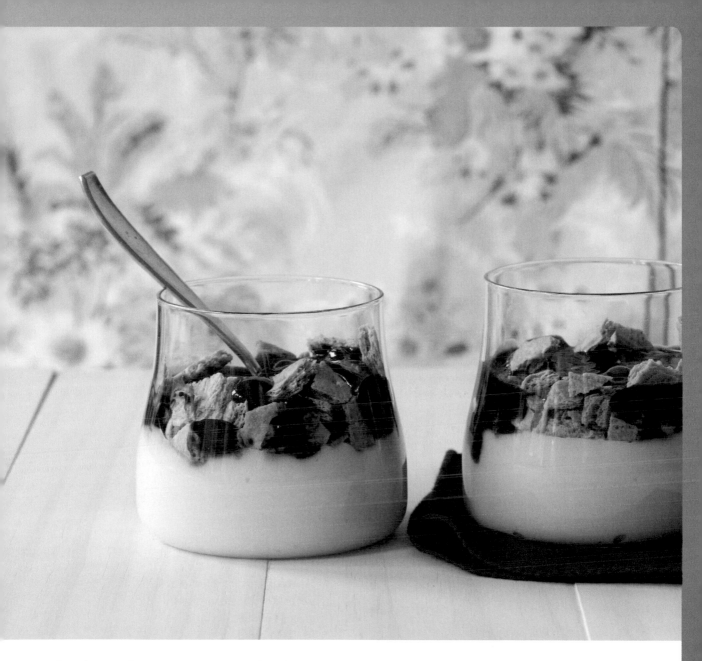

chocolate is velvety and melted. Top each pudding with a crumbled graham cracker square and 1 tablespoon of the melted chocolate sauce. Assemble right before serving so the chocolate doesn't harden.

---

nutrition information PER SERVING
185 calories ▪ 5 g protein ▪ 5 g total fat (3 g unsaturated, 2 g saturated) ▪ 65 mg cholesterol ▪ 30 g carbs ▪ 0.5 g fiber 22 g total sugar (4 g natural, 18 g added) ▪ 133 mg sodium

TASTY TWIST Save prep time by using store-bought low-fat vanilla pudding cups or prepare instant vanilla pudding mix using skim milk. You can also top these with 1 tablespoon of semisweet chocolate chips instead of melting the chocolate, or squirt on 1 tablespoon of store-bought chocolate sauce.

Junk Food

200 CALORIES

CHOCOLATE CUPCAKES WITH VANILLA FROSTING

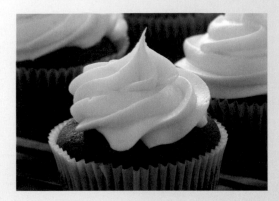

You can't beat the simplicity (and flavor) of store-bought cupcake mixes. But most call for two to three eggs and up to ½ cup of oil. Add the creamy canned frosting, and you're talking 200 calories and about 24 grams of sugar (roughly 6 teaspoons) per treat.

Here's a sweet strategy you can use to have your cake and eat it, too: The first few bites matter most, so I've found that downsizing your cupcake allows you to satisfy both your taste buds and waistline. Therefore, a set of mini-cupcake tins can be a smart investment for your kitchen.

Also, I have two secret ingredients to amp up the health factor while cutting calories. First, replace the oil and eggs with pureed black beans (yes, you read that right). Then, whip up your own nutrient-packed icing using avocado (trust me on this one—the color is green, but the taste is delicious).

Joy Food

70 CALORIES

MINI CHOCOLATE CUPCAKES WITH VANILLA FROSTING

makes 46 servings

Using black beans in place of oil and eggs is a simple way to health-ify boxed cake mixes. Think your taste testers will be scared off by the swap? I guarantee they'll never know (Hoda and Kathie Lee happily gobbled them up on the *Today* show without suspecting a thing).

Feel like having a second mighty mini? Double up guilt-free. You'll still be consuming far fewer calories and less sugar compared with the original, with 2 grams of fiber to boot.

MINI CUPCAKES
One 15.5-ounce can black beans, drained and rinsed
1 box dark chocolate cake mix

FROSTING
1 ripe avocado
⅛ teaspoon lemon juice
1 teaspoon vanilla extract
¼ teaspoon cream of tartar
1¾ cups confectioners' sugar
Cocoa powder (optional)

To make the mini cupcakes: preheat the oven to 350°F.

Puree the beans in a food processor or blender with 1 cup water until well blended. In a separate bowl, combine the cake mix with the pureed beans and mix well.

Line mini-cupcake tins with cupcake liners, and spoon the batter into them, filling the cups about halfway. Bake 10 to 12 minutes, or until a toothpick inserted into the center of a cupcake comes out clean.

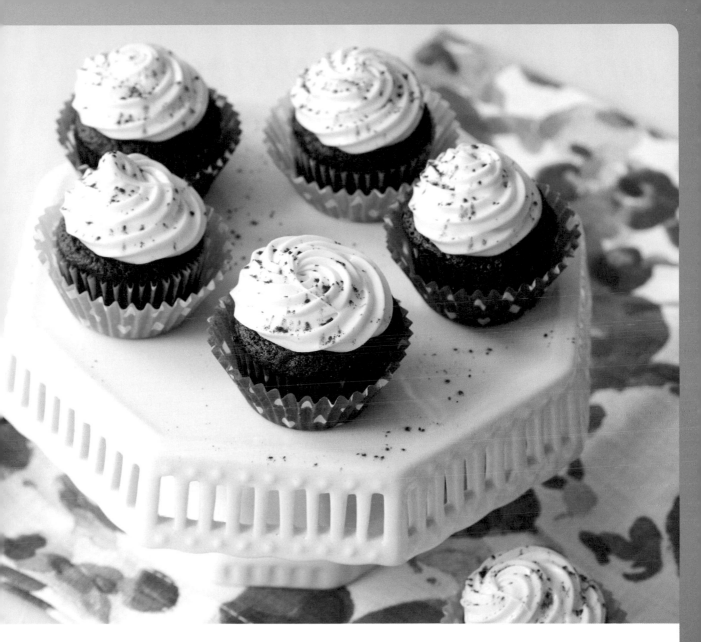

You can easily freeze any un-iced mini cakes, wrapped well, for up to 3 months. Defrost whenever you're craving something sweet.

To make the frosting: cut the avocado in half, remove the pit, and scoop out the meat.

Combine the avocado meat with the lemon juice, vanilla, and cream of tartar in a food processor or with a hand mixer. Mix until smooth, then add the confectioners' sugar, and mix well.

Top each mini cupcake with about 1 teaspoon of frosting. Or for a stiffer consistency, place the frosting in the refrigerator for a couple of hours before using it. For pretty presentation, garnish each mini with a dash of cocoa powder on top, if desired.

---

nutrition information PER SERVING
70 calories ▪ 1 g protein ▪ 1.5 g total fat (1 g unsaturated, 0.5 g saturated) ▪ 0 mg cholesterol ▪ 13 g carbs ▪ 1 g fiber 8 g total sugar (0 g natural, 8 g added sugar) ▪ 110 mg sodium

Junk Food

BROWNIES

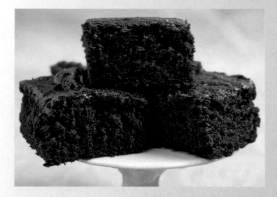

When you sink your teeth into a rich, chocolaty, fudgy coffee-shop brownie, the last thing you care about is calories, but sadly, they're still there—a whole lot of them. (And the fat and sugar, too.)

I'm not saying that you should bypass the brownie. That would be blasphemy. I'm just suggesting that you get a little creative when you make them at home, as I was with my recipe. Before you roll your eyes and flip to the next page, I strongly suggest you give it a shot. No one would ever suspect black beans. Yep, I went there. And I promise they're amazing.

> **CHOOSE IT TO LOSE IT** Swap your coffee-shop brownie for my slimmer spin once a week and, at the end of the year, you'll save more than 9,000 calories and drop up to 3 pounds (not to mention increase your fiber intake . . . pretty sweet for a treat).

Joy Food

BLACK BEAN BROWNIES

makes 20 servings

These brownies are a sneaky way to add a dose of nutrition into a yummy treat. I had *Today* show co-host Matt Lauer try a batch on the air, and while he was a skeptic at first, he was pleasantly surprised by the rich and fudgy taste. Score!

> One 15-ounce can black beans, drained and rinsed
> 1 box brownie mix
> 1 egg, beaten (optional)

After draining and rinsing, put the beans back into the can and add enough water to cover the beans. Put the beans and water into a blender and puree well.

Combine the bean puree with a standard box of brownie mix in a mixing bowl. Add the egg if you would like a softer, spongier consistency. Mix thoroughly and bake according to box directions.

---

nutrition information PER SERVING
120 calories ▪ 2 g protein ▪ 1 g total fat (1 g unsaturated, 0 g saturated) ▪ 0 mg cholesterol ▪ 27 g carbs ▪ 2 g fiber 16 g total sugar (0 g natural, 16 g added) ▪ 80 mg sodium

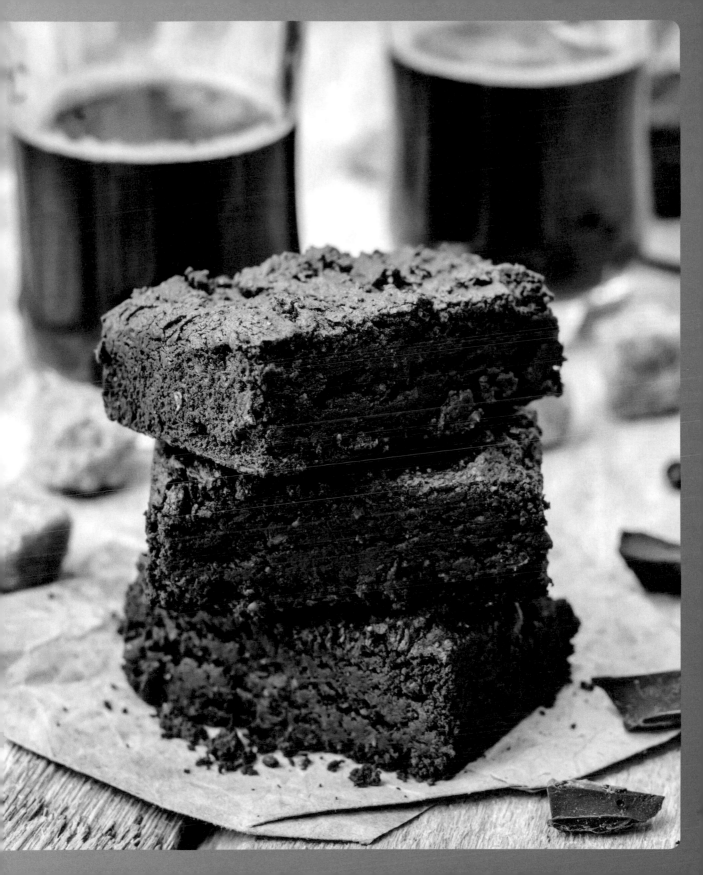

Junk Food

140 CALORIES

MARSHMALLOW TREATS

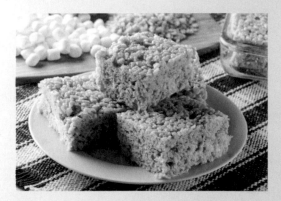

These treats, made with butter, puffed rice cereal, and marshmallows, aren't actually a bad choice if you're looking to satisfy the old sweet tooth. With only 140 calories per homemade square, you won't do much dietary damage.

However, I'm always looking for tasty ways to snip a few calories or squeeze in a few more fiber grams. That's why I was up for the challenge of health-ifying this family favorite. It was a tough one, but according to my kiddos—and nieces, nephews, and neighbors—I nailed it!

Joy Food

80 CALORIES

MARSHMALLOW POPCORN TREATS

makes 12 servings

The idea for this recipe came to me when I was staring at a box of cereal: Why not use popcorn instead? It's a whole grain and has a little more fiber than refined rice cereal. It also has more volume, so your treat will automatically be more slimming than the standard square. And by swapping typical stick butter for the whipped variety, I was able to cut a few more calories. That leaves a little extra room to top it off with a drizzling of melted chocolate, if you're looking for a more indulgent splurge. It's only 20 more calories per treat.

⅓   8

½ cup popcorn kernels or 6 cups air-popped or store-bought light popcorn

3 tablespoons whipped butter

4 cups mini marshmallows

¼ cup semisweet chocolate chips (optional)

Spray a 7 x 11–inch pan with nonstick oil spray and set aside.

Prepare 6 cups of plain popcorn in an air popper or use this microwave method: Place ¼ cup popcorn kernels in a brown paper lunch bag and fold the edge over 2 or 3 times to seal it. Microwave the bag on high for about 2 minutes or until the popping slows to 2 seconds between pops. Pour the popcorn into a large bowl and let it cool. Repeat the process with the remaining ¼ cup of popcorn kernels. (This method will likely yield more popcorn than you need; be sure to measure 6 cups before making treats.)

Melt the butter in large pan over low heat. Add the marshmallows and stir continuously until they melt and the mixture is well blended.

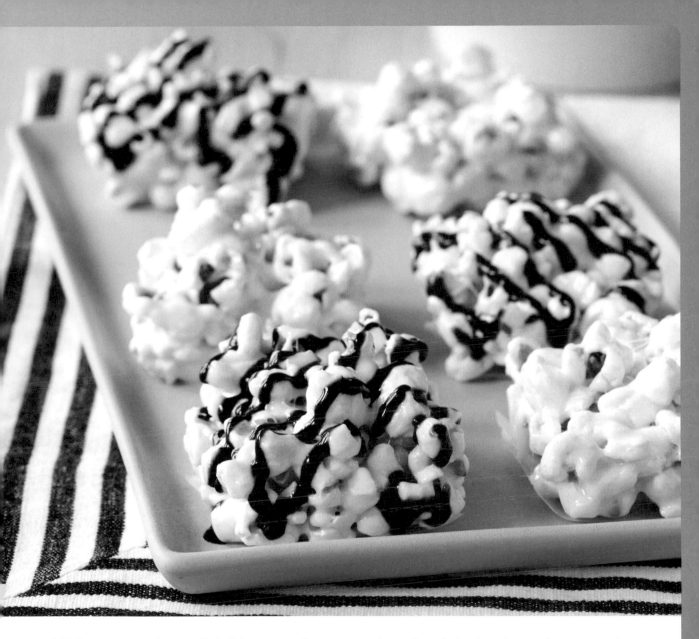

Add the popcorn and stir until all of the popcorn is covered and coated in melted marshmallows.

Pour the mixture into the prepared pan and press down to spread and shape. (Spray your hands with nonstick oil spray so the popcorn doesn't stick.)

Let the treats cool and harden.

If using the chocolate, melt the chocolate in the microwave by heating for 15 to 30 seconds at a time, stirring in between, until the chocolate is smooth and velvety. Or melt the chocolate on the stove top in a double boiler or saucepan over low heat. Drizzle the melted chocolate in any preferred design over the top of the marshmallow treats.

Cut into 12 squares and enjoy.

nutrition information PER SERVING
80 calories ▪ 1 g protein ▪ 2 g total fat (1 unsaturated, 1 g saturated) ▪ 5 mg cholesterol ▪ 15 g carbs ▪ 0.5 g fiber 9 g total sugar (0 g natural, 9 g added) ▪ 30 mg sodium

Junk Food

730 CALORIES

STRAWBERRY CHEESECAKE

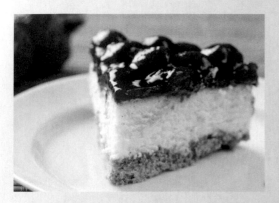

Cheesecake? Yes, please! Then, prepare for a body shock, no thanks to the fattening ingredients like butter, cream cheese, sugar, and sometimes sour cream. Sure, some versions might contain a bit of fruit, but don't let that fool you into thinking it's a good-for-you dessert selection. A single slice of strawberry cheesecake from a popular chain restaurant contains 730 calories. (To put that into perspective, you'd have to eat 182 strawberries to hit that number.)

Still, I understand that life is better with cheesecake, so I found a way for you to have your cake and eat it, too . . . well, sort of.

Joy Food

92 CALORIES

CHEESECAKE-STUFFED STRAWBERRIES

makes 10 servings

These bite-sized beauties contain just 23 calories a pop, which means you can enjoy a serving of four and still feel virtuous. It's the perfect portion of rich, creamy filling combined with the sweetness of strawberries—a win-win.

- 1 cup part-skim ricotta cheese
- 1 cup low-fat cottage cheese
- 2 egg whites
- ⅓ cup sugar
- 1 teaspoon lemon zest plus additional for garnish (optional)
- 1 teaspoon lemon juice
- 1 teaspoon vanilla extract
- ¼ teaspoon kosher salt or coarse sea salt
- 1 tablespoon cornstarch
- 40 strawberries

Preheat the oven to 300°F.

In a food processor, blend the ricotta cheese and cottage cheese until smooth.

Add the egg whites, sugar, lemon zest, lemon juice, vanilla, salt, and cornstarch, and pulse for a few seconds so everything comes together.

Liberally coat a 9-inch round pan with nonstick oil spray and pour the cheese mixture into the pan. Bake for 50 minutes. Remove the cheesecake from the oven and let it cool. (To cool more quickly, place the cheesecake in the freezer for about 15 minutes.)

While the cheesecake is cooling, wash the strawberries and slice off the tips to create a flat surface for the berries to stand on. Then, using a small knife, cut off the green stem and carve out a bit of the inner strawberry to make room to pipe in the cheesecake filling.

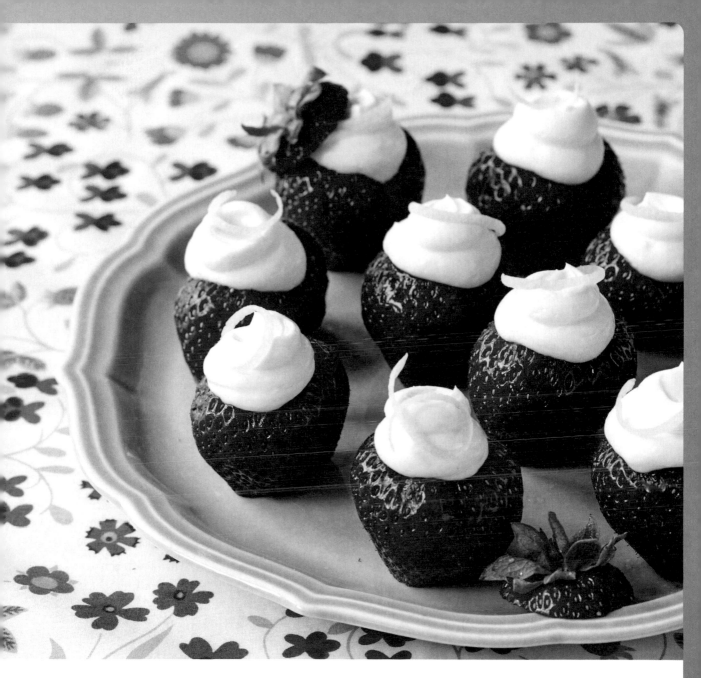

When the cheesecake has cooled, scoop it into a zip-top bag (all at once or in small batches), and push the cheesecake down toward one corner. Using a pair of scissors, cut a small hole in the bottom corner of the bag to create an opening for the cheesecake mixture to flow out. Squeeze the cheesecake filling into each strawberry, using approximately 2 to 3 teaspoons per berry. Garnish with the additional lemon zest, if desired.

nutrition information PER SERVING OF 4 STRAWBERRIES
92 calories ▪ 5.5 g protein ▪ 2 g total fat (0.5 unsaturated, 1.5 g saturated) ▪ 10 mg cholesterol ▪ 13.5 g carbs
1 g fiber ▪ 9.5 g total sugar (4 g natural sugar, 5.5 g added sugar) ▪ 138 mg sodium

Junk Food

400 CALORIES

PUMPKIN PIE

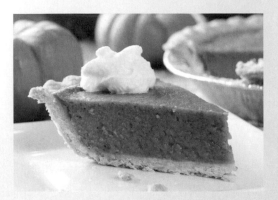

I love it when the temperature cools slightly and the leaves start to change color in the fall—that's a sign that one of my favorite veggies will start making its appearance in coffees, soups, and, yes, pies. Pumpkin pie is a family favorite in my house, but because of its high calorie cost (400 per average slice), we try to enjoy it sparingly.

Always up for a challenge, I took to my kitchen to find a way to lighten up the orange-orb treat. Success! You can enjoy this mini masterpiece any day of the week—no need to wait for Thanksgiving.

Joy Food

180 CALORIES

MINI PUMPKIN PIES

makes 6 servings

I shrunk traditional pumpkin pie into individual mini versions—a tasty, portion-controlled indulgence that will satisfy any craving without facing the temptation of seconds. The star ingredient, pumpkin, is rich in beta-carotene to nourish skin, protect your joints, and keep eyesight sharp. Go ahead and dig in.

    6 mini graham-cracker crusts
    1 cup 100% pumpkin puree
    ½ cup skim milk
    1 egg
    1 egg white
    ⅓ cup pure maple syrup
    ¾ teaspoon cinnamon plus additional for
        garnish (optional)
    ⅛ teaspoon nutmeg
    ⅛ teaspoon ginger
    1 pinch of kosher salt or coarse sea salt
    Canned whipped topping (optional)

Preheat the oven to 375°F. Arrange the crusts on a baking sheet.

In a large bowl, whisk together the remaining ingredients—except the whipped cream—until smooth. Divide the filling evenly between the 6 crusts. The crusts will be very full, and you may have some filling left over.

Bake the pies for 25 minutes, or until a toothpick inserted into the center of one comes out clean.

Cool the pies to room temperature. Garnish each pie with a dollop of whipped cream and sprinkle with the cinnamon, if desired.

---

nutrition information PER SERVING
180 calories ▪ 4 g protein ▪ 5 g total fat (2 g unsaturated, 3 g saturated) ▪ 31 mg cholesterol ▪ 29 g carbs ▪ 2 g fiber 19.5 g total sugar (2 g natural, 17.5 g added) ▪ 160 mg sodium

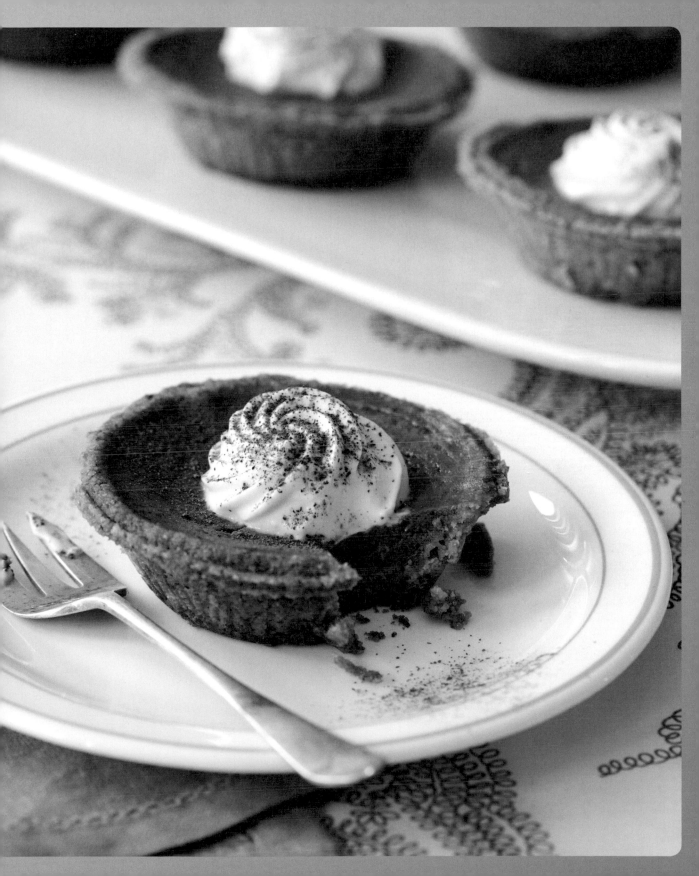

Junk Food

500 CALORIES

APPLE PIE

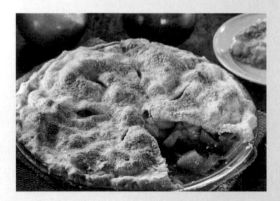

There's nothing quite like the smell (or taste) of homemade apple pie fresh from the oven. Top a slice with some ice cream, and it's like heaven on earth . . . plus a thunderstorm of calories, fat, and sugar. Sigh.

Good news: When it comes to this American staple, there are plenty of tricks to slim down your fix so you can enjoy it more regularly without the lousy aftermath. For example, slice off the outer crust and you'll automatically save yourself 100 calories. And when you're following a recipe, use supersweet apples like Fuji or Honeycrisp and reduce the sugar by about a quarter. Finally, try my apple-oatmeal combo, which delivers the same comforting flavors and is healthy enough to enjoy for breakfast.

> **CHOOSE IT TO LOSE IT** Trade in your traditional apple pie for this new and improved version once a week, and, by the end of the year, you'll slice more than 14,000 calories off your diet and potentially drop 4 pounds.

Joy Food

220 CALORIES

BAKED APPLE OATMEAL "PIE"

makes 4 servings

Satisfy your sweet tooth with this scrumptious, slimming dessert recipe that pairs delicious apples with fiber-rich oats and flavorful spices. Your kitchen will smell so amazing while this dish is cooking, the UPS man might just stick around after delivering a package, hoping to score a sample.

> 4 large apples
> 1 cup old-fashioned rolled oats
> ½ cup unsweetened applesauce
> 2 tablespoons honey
> 1 teaspoon vanilla extract
> ½ teaspoon cinnamon
> ½ teaspoon pumpkin pie spice
> 1 teaspoon fresh lemon zest (optional)
> 2 tablespoons raisins (optional)
> 2 tablespoons chopped walnuts (optional)

Preheat the oven to 350°F.

Rinse, core, and slightly hollow the apples, leaving the bottom of the apple intact to create a well for the filling. Place the apples in a pie pan. (Consider slicing off apple tops carefully and cooking them in the pie pan alongside apples. It makes for a pretty presentation when serving.)

In a medium bowl, combine the oats, applesauce, honey, vanilla, cinnamon, and pumpkin pie spice. Add the lemon zest, raisins, and/or chopped walnuts, if desired.

Fill each apple with the oat mixture until it is overflowing. Bake for 40 minutes, or until the sides of the apples are soft and easily pierced with a knife.

---

nutrition information PER SERVING
220 calories ▪ 3 g protein ▪ 2 g total fat (1.5 g unsaturated, 0.5 g saturated) ▪ 0 mg cholesterol ▪ 51 g carbs ▪ 7 g fiber 31 g total sugar (22.5 g natural, 8.5 g added) ▪ 0 mg sodium

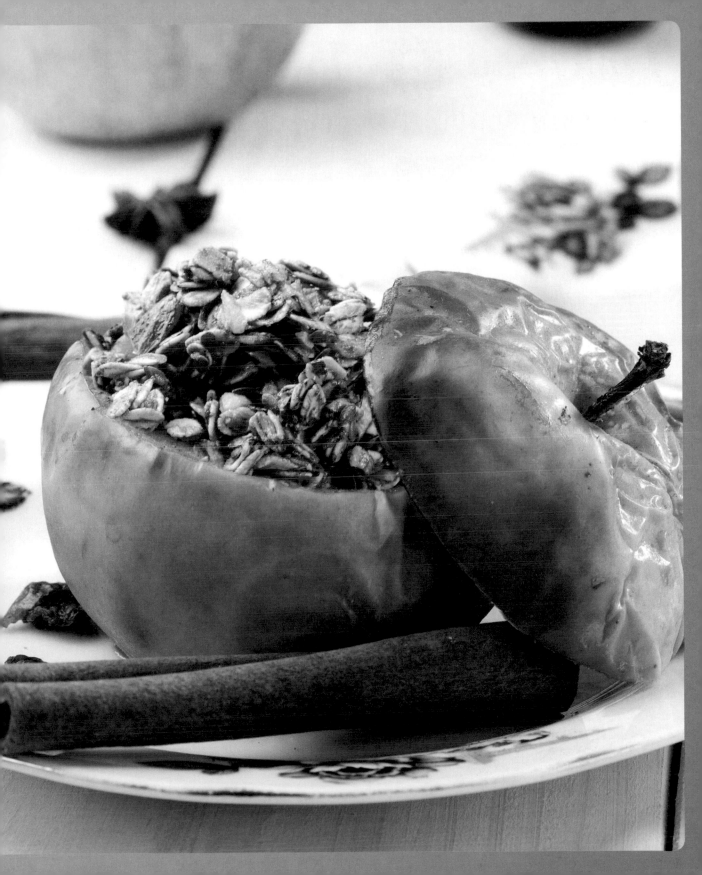

Junk Food

260 CALORIES

PUMPKIN PUDDING

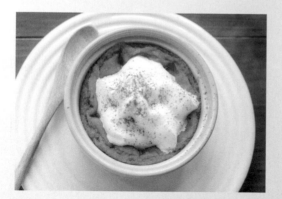

When it comes to pie, some people lust after the crust, while others say it's what's inside that counts. For me, I'm all about the filling, and this is particularly true for pumpkin pie. Which brings me to pumpkin pudding . . . I'm crazy for the creamy stuff. But because the decadent dessert is traditionally made with heavy ingredients, I set out to create a lightened-up alternative.

My new and improved Pumpkin Pudding is ridiculously easy to make and doesn't require any baking. The best part? You can enjoy the delicious seasonal treat any time of day, at any time of year. Grab your spoon.

Joy Food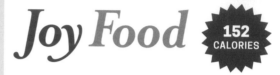

152 CALORIES

PUMPKIN PUDDING

makes 1 serving

My simple pudding makes a terrific quick breakfast or afternoon snack. The key ingredient is canned pumpkin puree, which is low in calories, high in fiber, and bursting with beta-carotene. And thanks to the yogurt, you'll get bone-strengthening calcium and a good amount of protein. Happy Thanksgiving—any day of the year.

> 6 ounces nonfat vanilla Greek or
> traditional yogurt
> ⅓ cup 100% pumpkin puree
> Dash of cinnamon
> 1 tablespoon toasted chopped almonds,
> walnuts, or pecans (optional)
> Pumpkin pie spice (optional)

Combine the yogurt, pumpkin, and cinnamon in a small bowl and mix until well combined. Top with the nuts and an extra sprinkle of the pumpkin pie spice or cinnamon, if desired.

---

nutrition information PER SERVING
152 calories • 18 g protein • 0 g total fat (0 g unsaturated, 0 g saturated) • 0 mg cholesterol • 20 g carbs • 2.5 g fiber 15 g total sugar (5.5 g natural, 9.5 g added) • 72 mg sodium

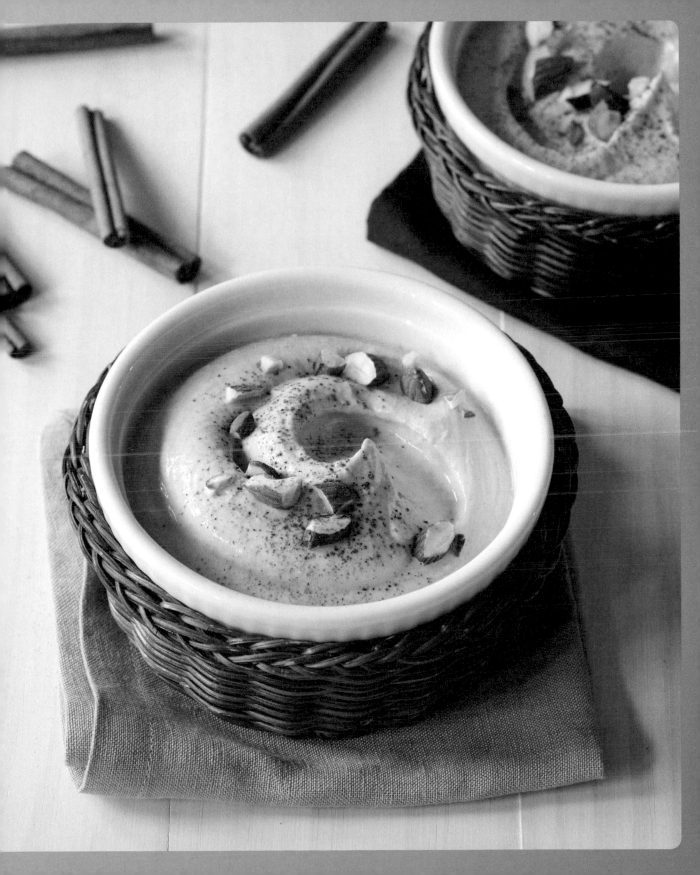

Junk Food

213 CALORIES

CHOCOLATE-MINT CANDIES

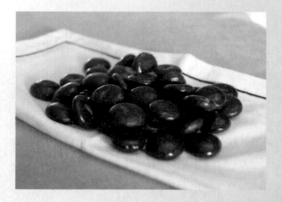

Who loves chocolate-mint candies? I sure do. While an occasional splurge is perfectly okay, it's important to know that these melt-in-your-mouth little guys pack a serious punch of fat and sugar (213 calories per 20 candies). In fact, the large box sold at the movie theater (it says three servings, but let's face it, we're eating the entire thing) crams in 510 calories, 9 grams of fat, and 96 grams sugar—that's 24 teaspoons of straight sugar.

I say indulge every once in a while on the real thing, and the rest of the time, whip up a batch of my skinny Chocolate-Mint Marshmallows. You'll get the flavors you crave without having to hop on the treadmill to burn off the damage.

Joy Food

145 CALORIES

CHOCOLATE-MINT MARSHMALLOWS

makes 1 serving

My version of the candy-store classic gives you that refreshing chocolate-mint combo without undoing your diet. Plus, you'll get a calcium kick for bone strength to boot. It's a perfect sweet treat to enjoy with your kids when you're hunkered indoors on a rainy day.

1 drop peppermint extract
1 low-fat chocolate pudding cup
20 mini marshmallows
Toothpicks

Mix the peppermint extract into a low-fat chocolate pudding cup. Poke the mini marshmallows with toothpicks and dip away.

---

nutrition information PER SERVING
145 calories ▪ 2 g protein ▪ 0 g total fat (0 g unsaturated, 0 g saturated) ▪ 0 mg cholesterol ▪ 33 g carbs ▪ 1 g fiber 24 g total sugar (8 g natural, 16 g added) ▪ 180 mg sodium

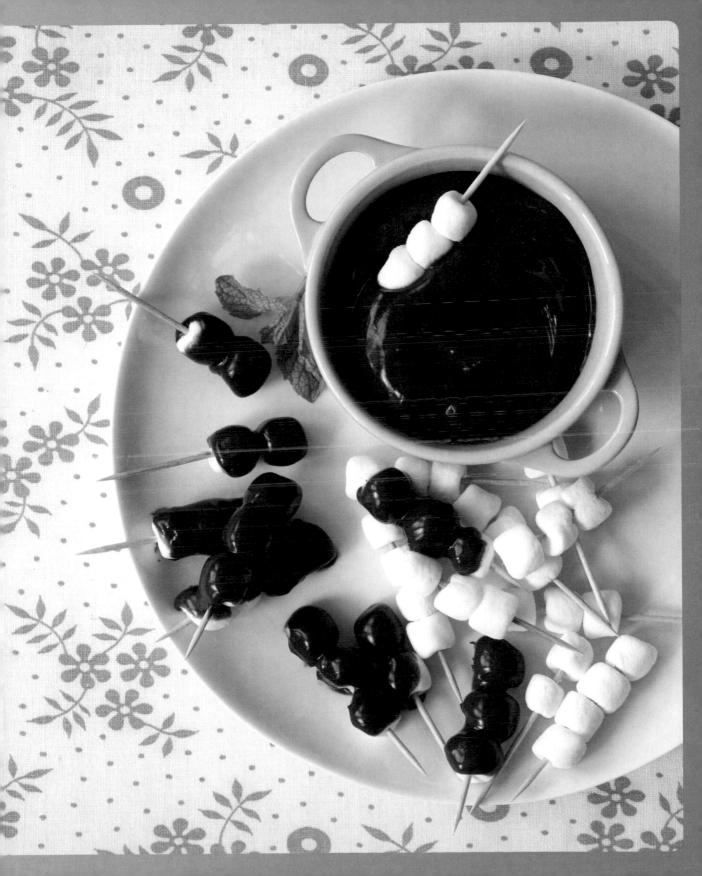

Junk Food

220 CALORIES

CHOCOLATE CRUNCH BARS

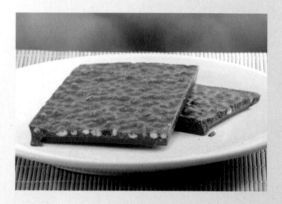

Remember the days of digging through your Halloween candy to eagerly find that chocolaty, crispy piece of deliciousness? Oh yeah, we all do.

Of course, I'm not going to pry away your favorite candy, at least not without offering up a healthier alternative first. Give my Chocolate Crunch Bars a shot—they're super-simple to make, and you'll score big points with friends and family.

Joy Food

148 CALORIES

CHOCOLATE CRUNCH BARS

makes 16 servings

Ready to turn two healthy ingredients into a delicious chocolate candy bar? Simply mix together melted dark chocolate with puffed brown-rice cereal, and you'll soon be the lucky recipient of a delicious dessert that's gluten-free and packed with goodness. Make it for your next party and don't expect any leftovers.

2 cups semisweet or dark chocolate chips
2 cups puffed brown-rice cereal

Line a baking sheet with parchment paper and set aside.

Melt the chocolate chips in a double boiler or saucepan on the stove top over low heat. Alternatively, you can melt the chocolate in the microwave by heating for 15 to 30 seconds at a time, stirring in between, until the chocolate is smooth and velvety.

Add the cereal into the melted chocolate and mix thoroughly.

Spread the mixture on the prepared baking sheet and place it in the fridge for at least 30 minutes. Once it's cool, cut it into bars or break it into irregular pieces and place them on a festive serving tray.

---

nutrition information PER SERVING
148 calories ▪ 2 g protein ▪ 9 g total fat (3 g unsaturated, 6 g saturated) ▪ 0 mg cholesterol ▪ 20 g carbs ▪ 2 g fiber 16 g total sugar (0 g natural, 16 g added) ▪ 10 mg sodium

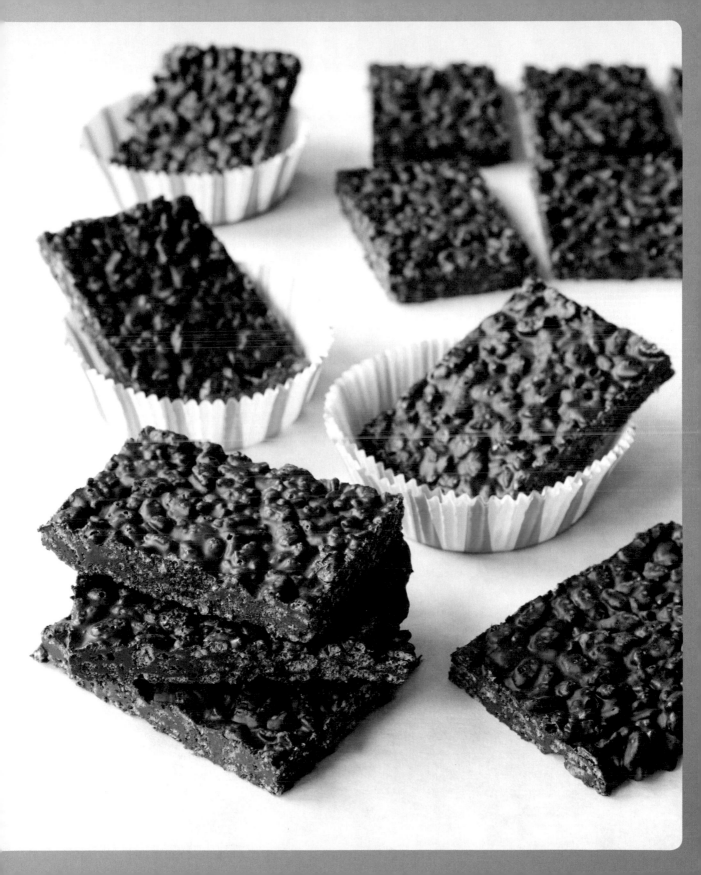

Junk Food

CHOCOLATE CHERRY CANDIES

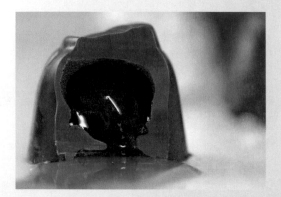

Chocolate cherry candies are a big seller on Valentine's Day and anniversaries. You can look past the calorie cost (about 80 per candy; and really, who eats just one?) and expense because it's an occasional splurge.

But why wait for a special event when you can enjoy an inexpensive and good-for-you alternative anytime you want? All you have to do is start with fresh fruit and dip it in a small amount of antioxidant-rich dark chocolate. It's a great way to get a taste of the good stuff without overpowering the fruit's naturally sweet flavor. Give my chocolate-dipped cherries a try to see what I'm talking about. And you don't have to limit yourself to just one—four of these are still better for you than one of those overly sweet, chocolate-smothered cherries you'll find in the store.

Joy Food

DARK CHOCOLATE CHERRIES

makes 10 servings

Portable, bite-sized, and fun to eat, cherries pack a potent nutritional punch. Rich in the antioxidant anthocyanin, these deliciously sweet gems help to fight inflammation and ease joint pain. Take advantage of them while you can—peak season is from May to August, so you'll likely find deals at your local supermarket when cherries are abundant. Dip 'em in melty dark chocolate, and you've created the ultimate power couple.

> 1 ounce dark chocolate (at least 60% cacao)
> or 2 tablespoons semisweet chocolate chips
> 10 fresh cherries with stems

Line a plate or baking sheet with parchment paper. Set aside.

Melt the chocolate in the microwave by heating for 15 to 30 seconds at a time, stirring in between, until the chocolate is smooth and velvety. Alternatively, melt the chocolate on the stove top using a double boiler or saucepan over low heat.

Dip each cherry into the melted chocolate so just the bottom third is covered in chocolate, and then place it on the prepared plate.

Cool the cherries in the refrigerator for 30 minutes or until the chocolate has hardened.

Enjoy . . . and be careful of the pits!

---

nutrition information PER SERVING
18 calories ▪ 0 g protein ▪ 1 g total fat (0.5 g unsaturated, 0.5 g saturated) ▪ 0 mg cholesterol ▪ 3 g carbs ▪ 0.5 g fiber 2.5 g total sugar (1.5 g natural, 1 g added) ▪ 0 mg sodium

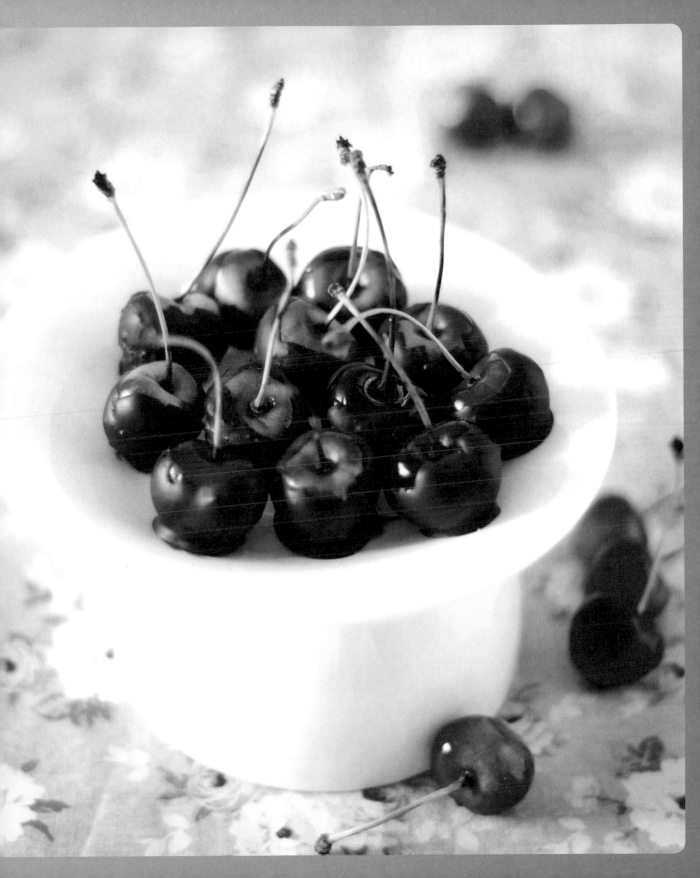

Junk Food

CHOCOLATE-COVERED POPCORN

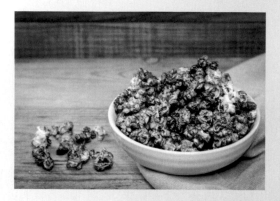

I've seen chocolate drizzled over all sorts of foods—bacon, pickles, even onions (don't ask!). But in my opinion, crunchy popcorn is a perfect base for the sweet topping. However, it's easy to go overboard, and some brands are way more chocolate than popcorn, which drives the calories sky high: 240 per cup, while a cup of plain air-popped popcorn has just 30 calories.

I might be a teensy bit biased, but my recipe strikes the right balance between the two ingredients. It keeps you satisfied without throwing your diet off the tracks.

Joy Food

DARK CHOCOLATE-COVERED POPCORN

makes 8 servings

Love popcorn? Love chocolate? Combine the two for a satisfying treat with the perfect mix of crunch and sweetness. It's a gourmet bite you can make right in your own kitchen . . . just be prepared to share!

- ½ cup popcorn kernels or 8 cups air-popped or store-bought light popcorn
- ½ cup dark or semisweet chocolate chips
- ½ teaspoon cinnamon
- ¼ teaspoon salt
- ¼ cup toasted slivered almonds (optional)

Line a large rimmed baking sheet with parchment or waxed paper and set aside.

Prepare 8 cups of plain popcorn in an air popper or use this microwave method: Place ¼ cup popcorn kernels in a brown paper lunch bag and fold the edge over 2 or 3 times to seal it. Microwave the bag on high for about 2 minutes or until the popping slows to 2 seconds between pops. Pour the popcorn into a large bowl and let it cool. Repeat the process with the remaining ¼ cup of popcorn kernels.

When the popcorn is ready, melt the chocolate in the microwave by heating for 15 to 30 seconds at a time, stirring in between, until the chocolate is smooth and velvety. Alternatively, melt the chocolate on the stove top in a double boiler or saucepan over low heat. Once the chocolate is smooth, remove it from the heat, add the cinnamon, and mix to incorporate thoroughly.

Pour the melted chocolate on the popcorn and toss to coat. Sprinkle on the salt and toss again to evenly distribute. Add the almonds, if desired, and toss one last time to incorporate.

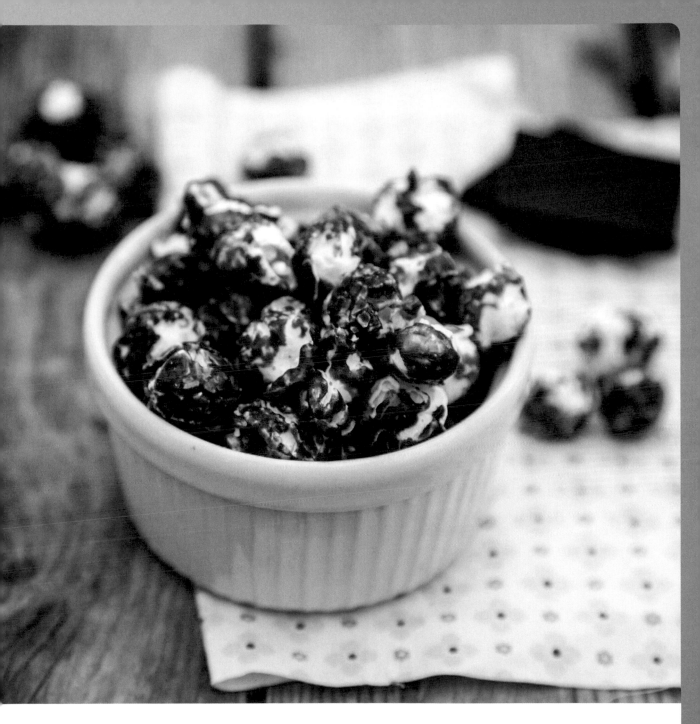

Spread the chocolate-popcorn mixture on the prepared sheet pan in an even layer, sprinkle it with some additional cinnamon, and refrigerate it until firm (at least 30 minutes).

Gently break the popcorn apart into clusters and serve.

nutrition information PER 1-CUP SERVING
100 calories ▪ 2 g protein ▪ 5 g total fat (2 g unsaturated, 3 g saturated) ▪ 0 mg cholesterol ▪ 15 g carbs ▪ 3 g fiber 8 g total sugar (0 g natural, 8 g added) ▪ 66 mg sodium

Junk Food

290 CALORIES

CHOCOLATE–PEANUT BUTTER CUPS

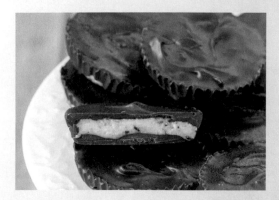

Chocolate and peanut butter are inarguably the perfect pair. In fact, the dynamic duo is, hands down, one of my favorite combos, but unfortunately homemade recipes tend to be north of 250 calories per decadent cup. So I've experimented with fun, creative, and more wholesome ways to couple these indulgent ingredients—and I think I hit upon something delicious that does the trick. I'm curious to hear what you think.

Joy Food

165 CALORIES

FROZEN CHOCOLATE–PEANUT BUTTER CUPS

makes 6 servings

Love packaged peanut butter cups? Whip up my insanely delicious, healthier version instead. Recruit the kids to give you a hand—the treats are a lot of fun to make. Plus, they're very rich, so you need only one to feel totally satisfied. Frozen bonus: they take a while to enjoy.

> 1 ripe banana
> ¼ cup creamy nut or seed butter (peanut, almond, sunflower seed, etc.)
> ½ teaspoon vanilla extract
> ½ cup dark chocolate chips, or 3-ounce dark chocolate bar
> ¼ cup unsweetened vanilla almond milk

In a small bowl, mix together the banana, nut butter, and vanilla. Mash everything together well and set aside.

Place 6 liners in a muffin tin and spray the liners liberally with nonstick oil spray. Silicone muffin liners work best, as it's easier to remove the chocolate when it's time to eat. Set the muffin tin aside.

In a saucepan, melt the chocolate and almond milk on medium heat, stirring constantly.

Once the chocolate is smooth, add a generous tablespoon of the mixture to the bottom of each muffin liner. Then stick the muffin tin in the freezer to firm up the chocolate (about 10 minutes).

Once the chocolate is firm, distribute the banana filling evenly among the muffin cups and spread the filling out with your fingers. Then split the remaining chocolate among the cups, using your fingers to spread each layer evenly.

Place the tin back in the freezer for at least 4 hours (overnight works best).

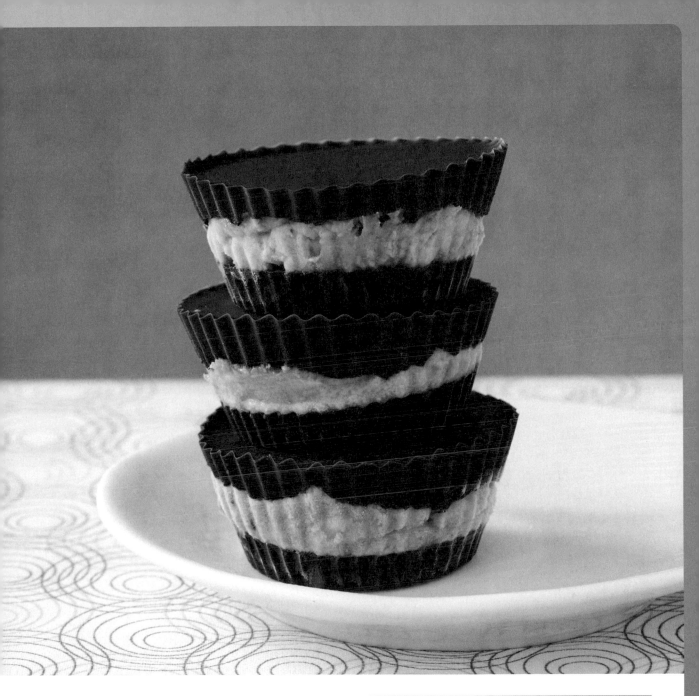

When you're ready to eat, pop each cup out of its liner and serve immediately!

---

nutrition information PER SERVING

165 calories ▪ 4 g protein ▪ 11.5 g total fat (7.5 g unsaturated, 4 g saturated) ▪ 0 mg cholesterol ▪ 13 g carbs ▪ 3 g fiber 6.5 g total sugar (2.5 g natural, 4 g added) ▪ 60 mg sodium

SERVE IT UP SLIM **Want to cut calories? Simply omit the peanut butter and enjoy a Frozen Chocolate-Banana Cup for only 90 calories.**

Junk Food

150 CALORIES

ITALIAN ICE

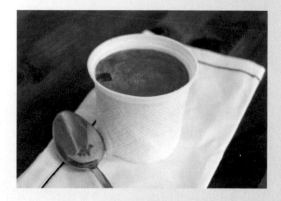

Although Italian ices are typically fat-free and lower in calories compared with ice cream, they are often jammed with added sugar (hello corn syrup!) and come packaged with artificial coloring and dyes. Consider this: a single-serve container of a popular brand contains 150 calories, 32 grams of sugar (that's 8 teaspoons), and controversial dyes (red no. 40, blue no. 1, and yellow no. 5) to ensure the color resembles the flavor. Not ideal.

Instead, try making your own tropical-flavored Italian ice—without a drop of added sugar. My refreshing homemade version will cool you down when the weather reaches record-breaking temperatures. Just two simple ingredients and 100 percent au naturel.

Joy Food

82 CALORIES

PIÑA COLADA ITALIAN ICE

makes 4 servings

This pineapple ice is a hot commodity in the Bauer house. My kids, nieces, and nephews swipe 'em from the freezer as fast as I make 'em. Using just two ingredients (so simple!), this tasty treat is brimming with piña colada flavor and take-me-to-the-tropics taste. I like to up the fun factor by freezing the ices in colorful ramekins and inserting small paper umbrellas after the mixture starts to solidify.

> One 20-ounce can crushed pineapple in its own juice
> 1 cup canned light coconut milk (see note)
> Small pineapple chucks (optional)

Pour the pineapple and juice into a pan and simmer over low heat for about 15 minutes to reduce some of the liquid. Add the coconut milk, stir to combine, and divide among 4 small ramekins or mugs. Place in the freezer for at least 4 hours or until solid. Garnish with small pineapple chucks, if desired.

Note: Because canned coconut milk tends to separate, make sure to shake the can well before you open it.

---

nutrition information PER ¾-CUP SERVING
82 calories ▪ 0 g protein ▪ 3 g total fat (1 g unsaturated, 2 g saturated) ▪ 0 mg cholesterol ▪ 13 g carbs ▪ 1 g fiber 12 g total sugar (12 g natural, 0 g added) ▪ 16 mg sodium

> **TASTY TWIST** If your crowd loves coconut, consider sprinkling on toasted coconut shreds right before serving. Or for an adult spin on this dessert, add 4 ounces of rum to the recipe before dividing into individual ramekins.

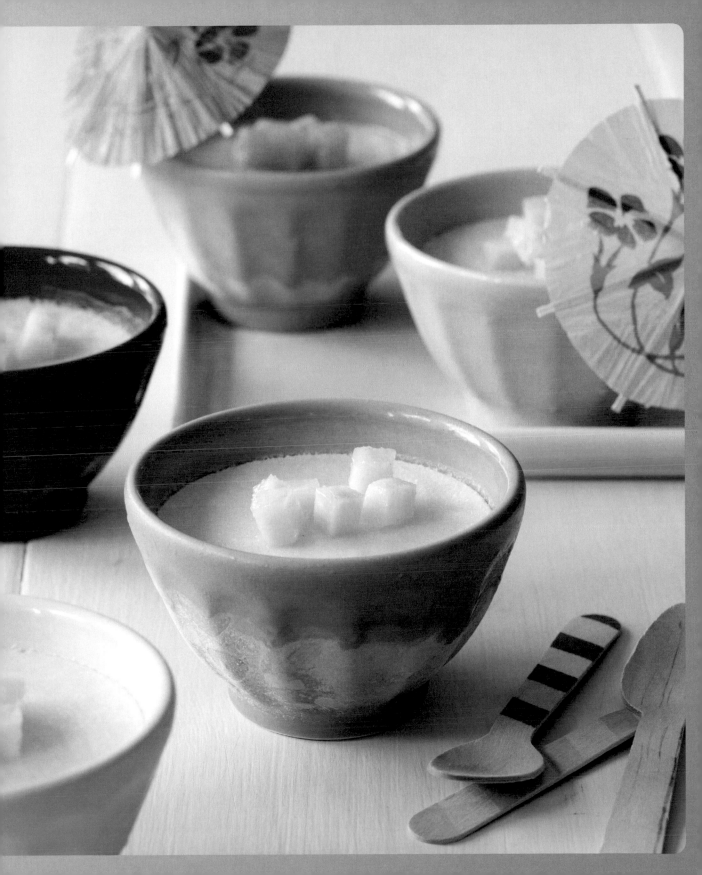

Junk Food

650 CALORIES

CHOCOLATE MILKSHAKE

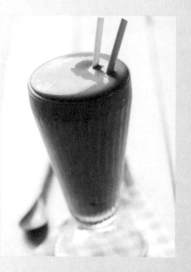

Chocolate milkshakes are a complete splurge. A small-sized sip will set you back about 650 calories. Order a large at a popular chain, and you'll slurp down more than 1,000—that exceeds some dinner entrées. Gulp!

But let's face it, there's no better way to satisfy your sweet tooth—milkshakes are creamy, chocolaty, and chilly. So how can you enjoy one without undoing your diet? Try my slimmed-down version by using light chocolate ice cream and unsweetened almond milk. I also add in half a banana for some extra creamy sweetness so you can sip stress-free.

> ▶ **CHOOSE IT TO LOSE IT** Make this milkshake switch once a week and you'll cut nearly 21,000 calories annually, which could translate to a loss of about 6 pounds in a year.

Joy Food

250 CALORIES

CHOCOLATE MILKSHAKE

makes 1 serving

This easy chocolate milkshake will satisfy even the biggest sweet tooth without sending you into calorie overload. (Trust me, it has been tested a million times by yours truly.) And while your taste buds rejoice, you'll feel good knowing that your body receives two heart-healthy ingredients: potassium-rich banana and flavanol-filled cocoa powder. It's a dessert with benefits.

½ cup unsweetened vanilla almond milk
¾ cup light chocolate ice cream
½ ripe banana
1 teaspoon unsweetened cocoa powder
Canned whipped topping
1 teaspoon chocolate shavings or mini chocolate chips (optional)

Add all the ingredients except the whipped topping and chocolate shavings to a blender and process until smooth and frothy. Finish off with a generous squirt of whipped topping. Add the chocolate, if desired, for only 15 extra calories.

---

nutrition information PER SERVING
250 calories ▪ 6 g protein ▪ 7 g total fat (3 g unsaturated, 4 g saturated) ▪ 20 mg cholesterol ▪ 41 g carbs ▪ 2 g fiber 26 g total sugar (16 g natural, 10 g added) ▪ 174 mg sodium

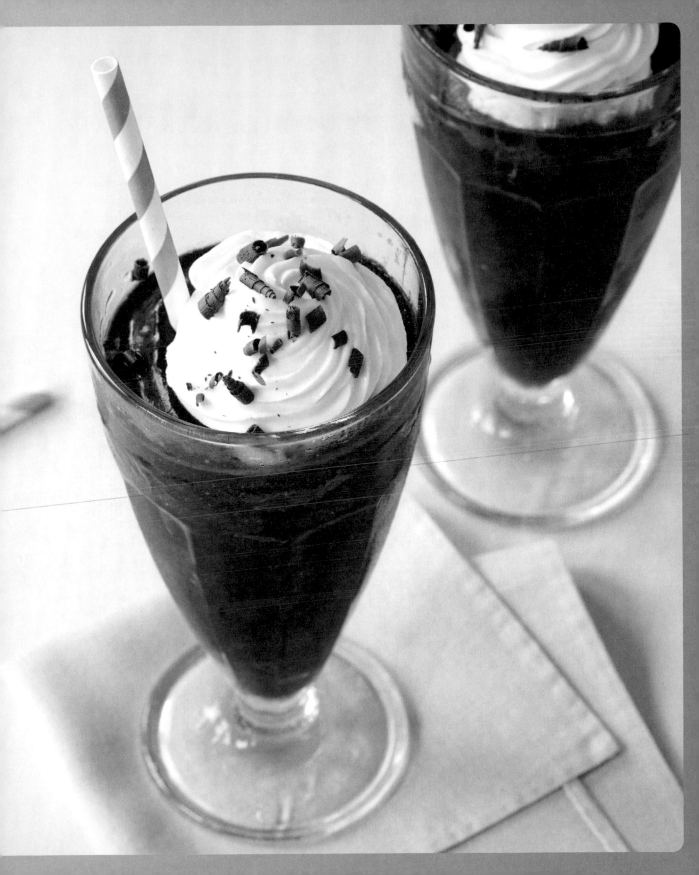

Junk Food

530 CALORIES

VANILLA MILKSHAKE

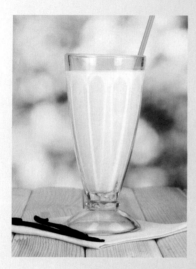

The rich and creamy flavor of a vanilla shake is to die for. And while the classic recipe calls for just two simple ingredients—vanilla ice cream and whole milk—in most instances, the decadent duo will pump your system with more than 500 calories. It also delivers a fair share of saturated fat and about 63 grams (that's 16 teaspoons) of sugar. It's a delish, but chaotic, combo.

Save the real deal for an occasional treat, and enjoy my skinny rendition for all the other times you need a fix.

Joy Food

120 CALORIES

VANILLA MILKSHAKE

makes 1 serving

This slimming, nondairy vanilla milkshake delivers natural sweetness and creaminess for only 120 calories. Simply toss four ingredients (plus a few ice cubes) into the blender and press a button—that's it. Then kick back and slurp your no-sugar-added fabulous and frothy beverage.

- ½ ripe banana, peeled and frozen
- ½ cup frozen pineapple
- ½ cup unsweetened vanilla almond milk
- 1 teaspoon vanilla extract
- 3 to 5 ice cubes

Add all the ingredients to a blender and process until smooth and frothy.

---

nutrition information PER SERVING
120 calories ▪ 1.5 g protein ▪ 1.5 g total fat (1.5 g unsaturated, 0 g saturated) ▪ 0 mg cholesterol ▪ 25 g carbs ▪ 3 g fiber
15 g total sugar (15 g natural, 0 g added) ▪ 90 mg sodium

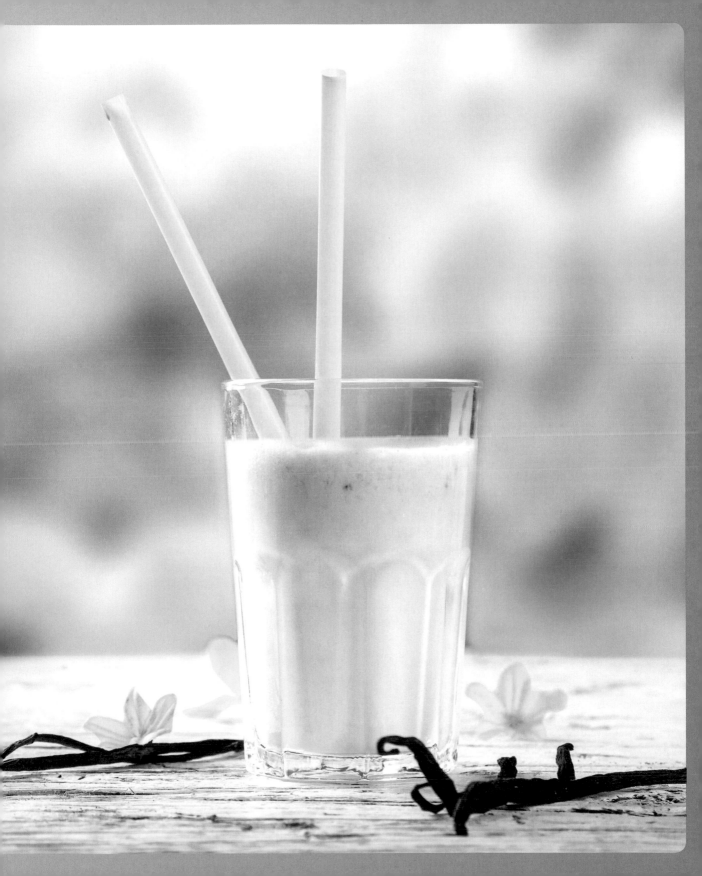

Junk Food

VANILLA ICE CREAM

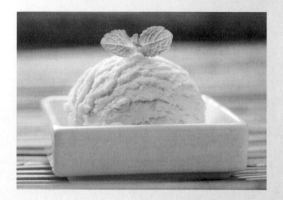

A chilly treat is a great way to beat the heat, but a measly ½-cup scoop of premium store-bought ice cream can sock you with at least 200 calories—and a whole lot of saturated fat and added sugar. Double or triple that amount and the calorie count starts to soar.

Admittedly, I could never live without ice cream, and every once in a while, I'm certainly down for a scoop (or two) of vanilla topped with all sorts of fixin's. As for my ice cream urges in between? I found an easy way to satisfy cravings using one healthful ingredient—bananas. Give my "nice" cream recipe a try, and I think you'll be hooked.

Joy Food

BANANA ICE CREAM
makes 3 servings

I love this nondairy frozen dessert option because it's made of pure, whole fruit (good old bananas) with no added sugar. Using ripe bananas is key to making it sweet and creamy. Be sure to try the peanut-butter variation, too—it's out-of-this-world delicious.

> 4 large ripe bananas
> Splash of milk (unsweetened vanilla almond milk, light coconut milk, soy milk, or skim milk) (optional)

Peel the bananas and cut them into 1-inch rounds. Place the bananas in a freezer bag and freeze them for at least 3 hours.

Place the banana slices in the bowl of a food processor. (If your banana slices have been in the freezer for longer than a day, it's best to let them thaw in the food processor bowl for about 15 minutes.)

Puree the bananas until they are completely smooth and no frozen chunks remain. If the bananas are too hard to blend, add a splash of milk for easier blending.

Scoop the ice cream into small bowls and serve immediately or cover in plastic wrap and freeze. If you're saving the ice cream for a later time, remove the bowls from the freezer about 5 minutes before serving the treat.

---

nutrition information PER ½-CUP SERVING
140 calories ▪ 2 g protein ▪ 0.5 g total fat (0.5 unsaturated, 0 g saturated) ▪ 0 mg cholesterol ▪ 36 g carbs ▪ 4 g fiber 19 g total sugar (19 g natural, 0 g added) ▪ 0 mg sodium

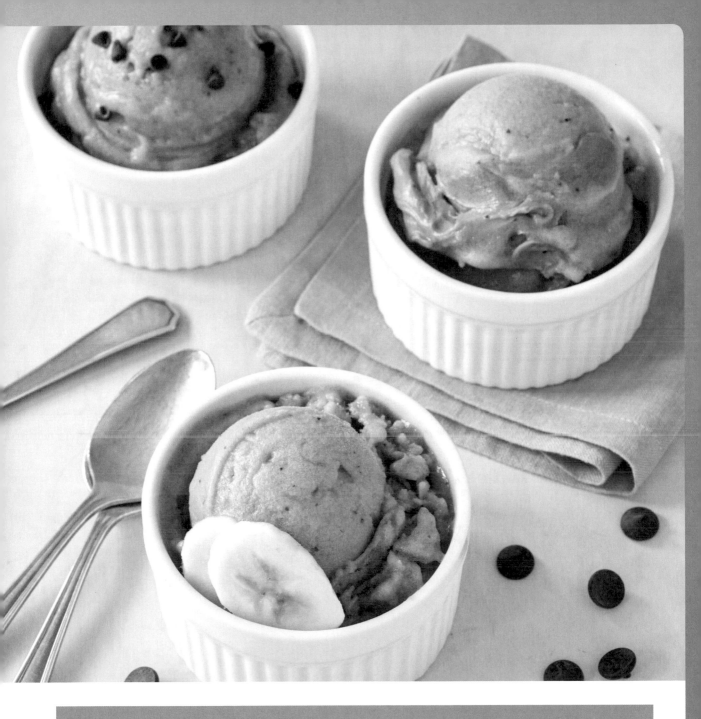

TASTY TWIST Top your Banana Ice Cream with 1 teaspoon of semisweet chocolate chips for only 25 extra calories. Or make PB-banana ice cream for a delicious taste sensation. To do this, add 2 tablespoons of natural peanut butter to the food processor after the bananas have been pureed. Puree for a few seconds longer to combine. Serve immediately or freeze for future (200 calories).

Junk Food

200 CALORIES

CHOCOLATE ICE CREAM

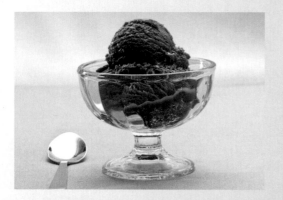

Vanilla or chocolate: What's your favorite ice cream flavor? Vanilla usually edges out chocolate as America's preferred pick, but most people I know scream for chocolate . . . with chocolate sauce . . . and chocolate sprinkles . . . and chocolate chips . . . and crushed chocolate cookies. That's a chocolotta heaven.

Unfortunately, the creamy-dreamy dessert comes at a steep calorie cost: a ½-cup scoop averages about 200 calories (that's 400 calories for a typical full-cup portion). Add 45 calories per tablespoon of sprinkles, 55 calories per tablespoon of fudge, 70 calories per tablespoon of chips, and before you know it, your belt buckle is busting and your insides are going cocoa-loco.

But life *is* better with chocolate. So I shut myself in my kitchen and wouldn't let myself out until I perfected a lighter and healthier option.

Joy Food

95 CALORIES

CHOCOLATE ICE CREAM

makes 6 servings

This chocolaty treat requires just five ingredients, has no added sugar, and contains about half the calories of ice cream parlor varieties. It's also dairy-free (though you can use cow's milk in place of coconut milk), and you can customize it based on what you like: add berries, chocolate chips, sprinkles, a little nut butter. It's all good.

> 4 ripe bananas
> ½ cup unsweetened cocoa powder
> ¼ cup unsweetened coconut milk beverage
> ½ teaspoon vanilla extract
> Pinch of salt

Peel and cut the bananas into 1-inch rounds. Place the bananas in a freezer bag and freeze them for at least 3 hours.

Right before you're ready to make the ice cream, whisk together the cocoa powder, coconut milk, and vanilla in a small bowl.

If your banana slices have been in the freezer for longer than a day, it's best to let them thaw in the food processor bowl for about 15 minutes. Place the frozen bananas, chocolate mix, and salt in a food processor and blend well, stopping to scrape down the sides often to get a smooth, even consistency.

Scoop the ice cream into small bowls and serve immediately or cover in plastic wrap and freeze. If you're saving the ice cream for a later time, remove the bowls from the freezer about 5 minutes to slightly thaw before serving the treat.

---

nutrition information PER ½-CUP SERVING
95 calories ▪ 2 g protein ▪ 1 g total fat (1 g unsaturated, 0 g saturated) ▪ 0 mg cholesterol ▪ 22 g carbs ▪ 3.5 g fiber 9.5 g total sugar (9.5 g natural, 0 g added) ▪ 20 mg sodium

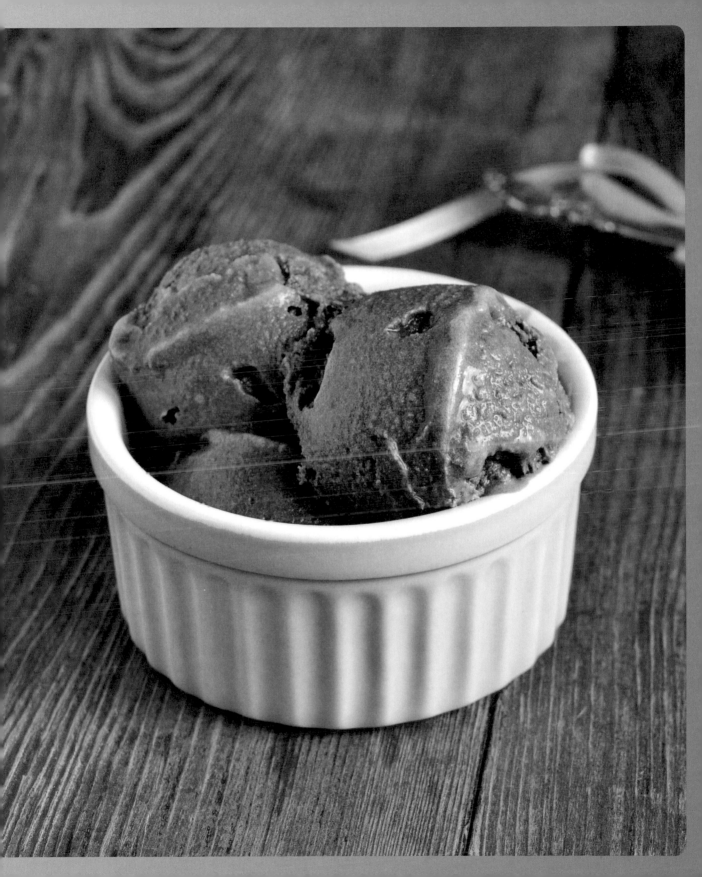

Junk Food

230 CALORIES

MINT CHOCOLATE CHIP ICE CREAM

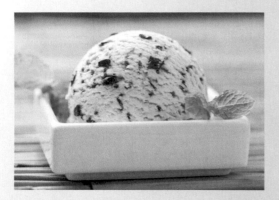

It's green, it's minty-licious . . . and it's fattening. Most popular brands of indulgent mint chocolate chip ice cream pack about 230 calories and 23 grams of sugar (that's almost 6 teaspoons) per scoop. I admit, it's a well-worth-the-calories occasional splurge.

But if you're looking to savor the flavor on a more regular basis, I have a smarter idea: my slimming take on this dessert is refreshingly minty while delivering almost 4 grams of filling fiber. Pretty darn cool for a frozen treat.

Joy Food

138 CALORIES

MINT CHOCOLATE CHIP ICE CREAM

makes 6 servings

If you're crazy for mint chip, you'll definitely want to try this skinny rendition. Full of refreshing minty flavor, this "nice" cream recipe is a breeze to toss together and provides an impressive amount of fiber. I originally created it for Carson Daly, but it now makes a daily appearance in my kitchen.

> 4 ripe bananas
> ½ cup unsweetened cocoa powder
> ¼ cup skim milk
> ½ teaspoon vanilla extract
> Pinch of salt
> Mint extract
> ¼ cup semisweet chocolate chips

Peel and cut the bananas into 1-inch rounds. Place the bananas in a freezer bag and freeze for at least 3 hours.

In a small bowl, whisk together the cocoa powder, milk, and vanilla.

If your banana slices have been frozen for longer than a day, let them thaw for about 15 minutes. Place the frozen bananas, chocolate mixture, and salt in a food processor and blend well, stopping to scrape down the sides often to get a smooth, even consistency. Add a drop of mint extract to the ice cream, blend, and taste. For a more intense mint flavor, increase the mint a drop at a time until you achieve the desired taste. Finally, add the chocolate chips into the ice cream and stir by hand until they're mixed throughout.

Scoop the ice cream into single-serving bowls and serve immediately or cover in plastic wrap and freeze. If you're saving these for a later time, remove the bowls from the freezer about 5 minutes before serving.

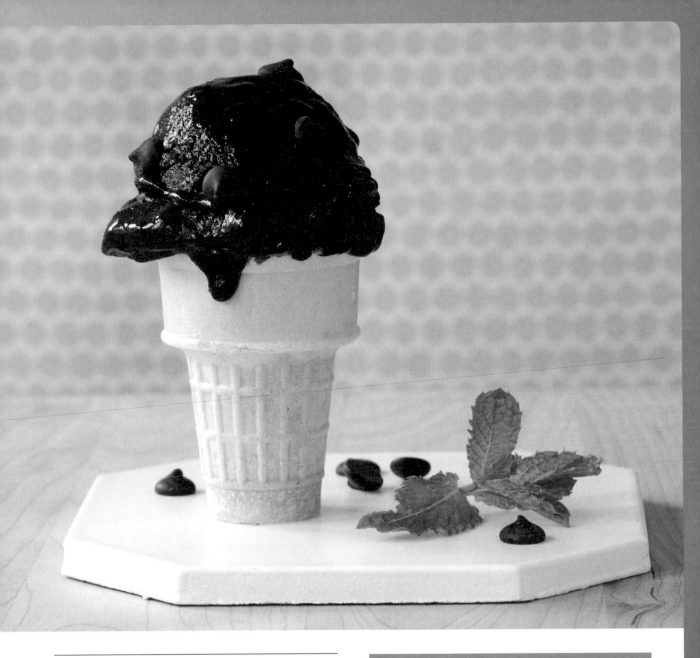

nutrition information PER ½-CUP SERVING

138 calories • 3 g protein • 4 g total fat (2 g unsaturated,
2 g saturated) • 0 mg cholesterol • 26 g carbs • 4 g fiber
14 g total sugar (9 g natural, 5 g added) • 28 mg sodium

> **TASTY TWIST** Make a Mint Chocolate
Chip Ice Cream Sandwich: scoop about ¼ cup
ice cream between two chocolate graham
cracker squares, gently press down on the
top piece to spread out the ice cream and
secure the sandwich, cover in plastic wrap,
and place in the freezer for at least 1 hour or
until it firms up. Enjoy for only 130 calories.

Junk Food

250 CALORIES

NEAPOLITAN ICE CREAM SANDWICH

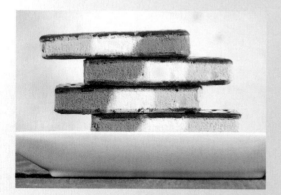

I scream, you scream, we all scream when we see the calorie counts of ice cream products. Sandwich that velvety goodness in between two chocolate cookies and it typically means diet derailment.

Not necessarily. My lightened-up ice cream sandwich, which features creamy vanilla, sweet cherries, and rich chocolate, contains just 145 calories. How much do you love me?!

Joy Food

145 CALORIES

CHERRY-VANILLA-CHOCOLATE ICE CREAM SANDWICH

makes 1 serving

Here's a delicious frozen treat that combines the fabulous flavors of chocolate, vanilla, and supersweet cherries. These ice cream sammies could not be easier to throw together . . . and they come out looking adorable. Whip up a batch and indulge guilt-free.

> ¼ cup light vanilla ice cream or frozen yogurt
> 6 frozen pitted cherries
> 1 chocolate graham cracker sheet,
>   broken in half

Soften the light vanilla ice cream and stir in the frozen cherries. (Alternatively, you can pulse and puree the frozen cherries in a food processor and then stir them throughout the softened ice cream to get a more even distribution.)

Scoop the ice cream between the chocolate graham cracker squares.

Put the sandwich in the freezer and let it set at least 1 hour.

---

nutrition information PER SERVING
145 calories ▪ 2.5 g protein ▪ 3 g total fat (2 g unsaturated, 1 g saturated) ▪ 5 mg cholesterol ▪ 28 g carbs ▪ 1.5 g fiber 18 g total sugar (10 g natural, 8 g added) ▪ 120 mg sodium

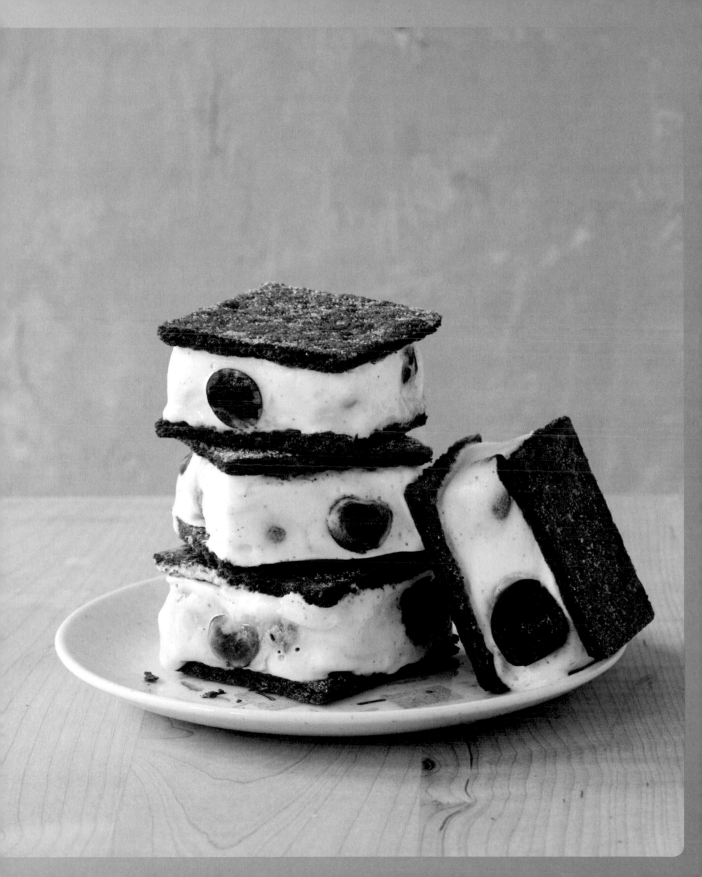

Junk Food

150 CALORIES

MANGO SORBET

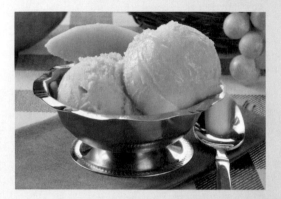

Craving a chilly treat but don't want all the calories and fat of ice cream? Sorbet is often a smart option. But many store-bought brands contain lots of added sugar.

My version contains no added sugar and has less than *half* the calories of popular brands. Plus, it's a snap to make.

Joy Food

64 CALORIES

MANGO-STRAWBERRY SORBET

makes 3 servings

Forget long lists of ingredients with names you can't even pronounce. This recipe contains just four items, three of which are produce. The result is delicious, simple, and only 64 calories per serving. It's the perfect dessert on a hot, summer day—chilly, light, and totally refreshing. My friends and family devour it!

> 1½ cups frozen mango chunks or 1 mango, peeled and diced
> 3 to 4 large strawberries, halved (approximately 1 cup)
> ¾ cup unsweetened coconut milk beverage
> 5 to 6 mint leaves (optional)

Combine all the ingredients in a blender and process until smooth.

Divide the mixture evenly among 3 bowls and freeze until firm, about 3 hours.

---

nutrition information PER ½-CUP SERVING
64 calories ▪ 1 g protein ▪ 1.5 g total fat (0.5 g unsaturated, 1 g saturated) ▪ 0 mg cholesterol ▪ 13 g carbs ▪ 2 g fiber 10.5 g total sugar (10.5 g natural, 0 g added) ▪ 0 mg sodium

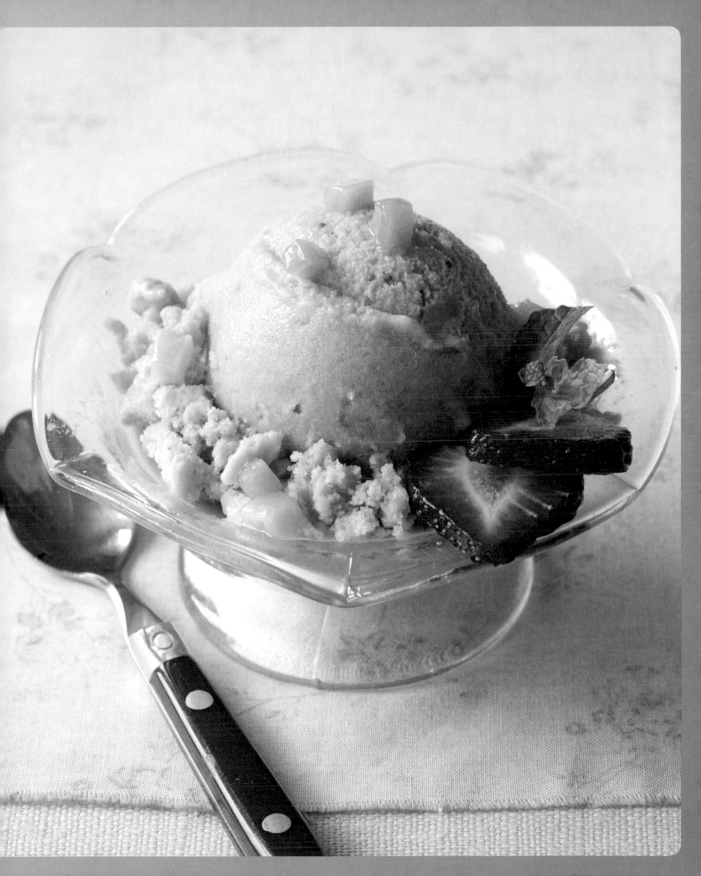

Junk Food

60 CALORIES

CHERRY ICE POPS

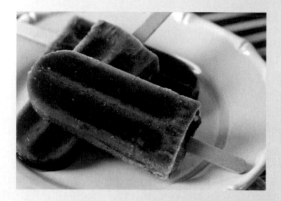

Cherry ice pops aren't a terrible choice when it comes to the calories, but they're made up almost entirely of sugar, so they're no bargain nutrition-wise. Plus, look closely at the ingredients list—many brands contain dyes to give their pops a nice, bright red color.

Whipping up your own wholesome, natural, and great-tasting pops right at home couldn't be any easier. It's foolproof, really. I made these cherry-pineapple creations especially for Hoda Kotb on the *Today* show when she swore off sugar for 10 long days. Hoda flipped for them, and I think you will, too.

Joy Food

40 CALORIES

CHERRY-PINEAPPLE POPS

makes 4 servings

Why go for store-bought when you can have homemade? Make a healthier version in your own kitchen using this simple recipe. It features three fiber-rich, naturally sweet fruits that create a flavorful ice pop for only 40 calories. Good to the last lick.

1 cup fresh or frozen pineapple
½ cup sweet, pitted fresh or frozen cherries
¼ cup unsweetened vanilla almond milk
½ cup sliced fresh or frozen strawberries

If you're using frozen fruit, let it thaw.

Combine all the ingredients in a food processor and blend until smooth.

Pour ½ cup of the mixture into 4 ice pop molds, and place them in the freezer for at least 4 hours, or until solid.

---

nutrition information PER SERVING
40 calories ▪ 1 g protein ▪ 0 g total fat (0 g unsaturated, 0 g saturated) ▪ 0 mg cholesterol ▪ 10 g carbs ▪ 1.5 g fiber
7 g total sugar (7 g natural, 0 g added) ▪ 10 mg sodium

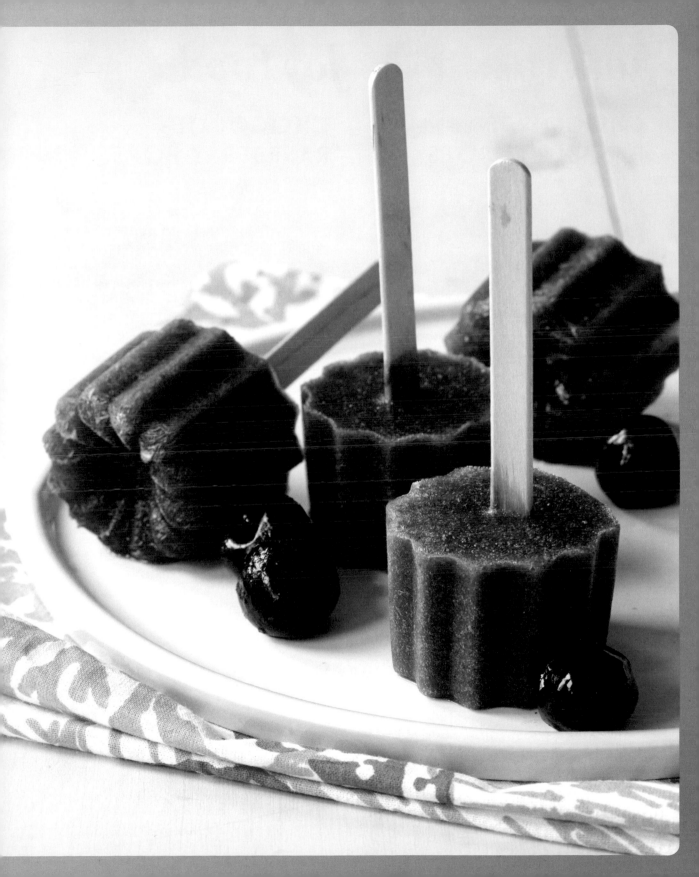

Junk Food

CHOCOLATE-RASPBERRY POPS

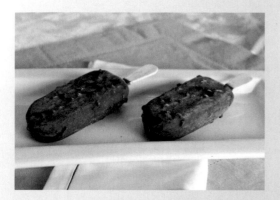

Heaven on a stick . . . that's what chocolate raspberry pops are. They are rich and creamy, sweet and indulgent, but on average, they're also 270 calories and contain about 20 grams of sugar, more than many of us can regularly afford to spend on a sweet treat.

I whipped up a batch of pops that mimic the flavor using just five simple ingredients. For only 90 calories and 3.5 grams of filling fiber, you can now enjoy this chocolate-raspberry remake whenever you feel like it.

Joy Food

CHOCOLATE-RASPBERRY POPS

makes 6 servings

Made with naturally sweet produce—frozen bananas and antioxidant-rich raspberries—these chilly pops are fresh, fiber filled, and loaded with fruity flavor. Each treat also delivers a dose of flavanol-packed cocoa powder. If you are avoiding dairy, swap in light coconut milk or unsweetened vanilla almond milk.

- 4 ripe bananas
- ½ cup unsweetened cocoa powder
- ¼ cup skim milk
- ½ teaspoon vanilla extract
- Pinch of salt
- 4 tablespoons fresh or frozen raspberries

Peel and cut the bananas into 1-inch rounds. Place the bananas in a freezer bag and freeze them for at least 3 hours.

In a small bowl, whisk together the cocoa powder, milk, and vanilla.

If your banana slices have been in the freezer for longer than a day, it's best to let them thaw in the food processor bowl for about 15 minutes. Place the frozen bananas, chocolate mix, and salt in a food processor and blend well, stopping to scrape down the sides often to get a smooth, even consistency.

Gently mix the raspberries into the ice cream with a spoon (do not puree). Pour about ½ cup of the mixture into each of 6 ice pop molds. Freeze for at least 5 hours or overnight. Enjoy!

nutrition information PER SERVING
90 calories ▪ 2.5 g protein ▪ 1 g total fat (1 g unsaturated, 0 g saturated) ▪ 0 mg cholesterol ▪ 20 g carbs ▪ 3.5 g fiber 9 g total sugar (9 g natural, 0 g added) ▪ 25 mg sodium

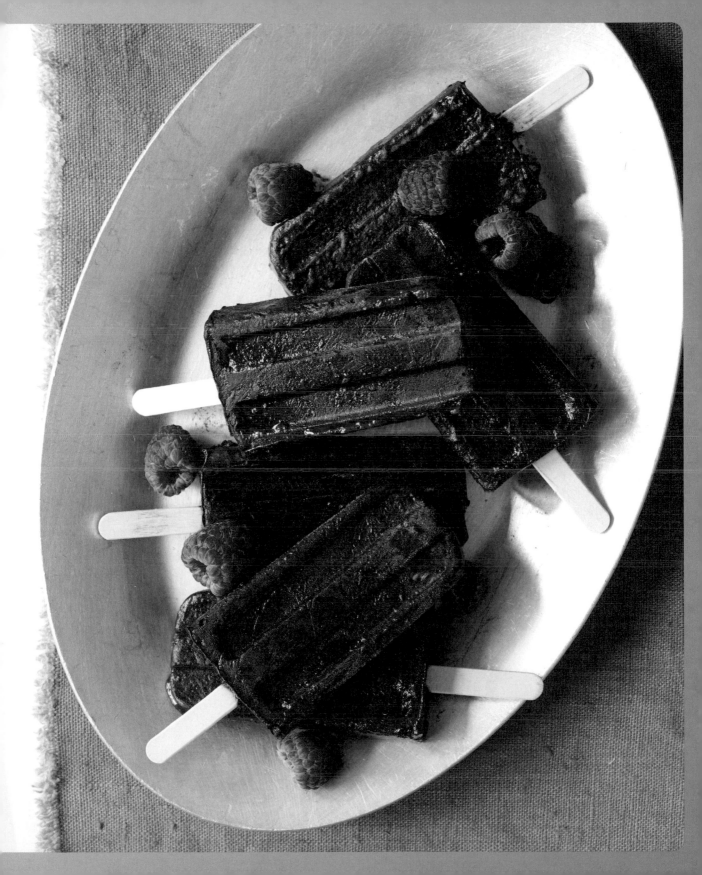

Junk Food

60 CALORIES

CLASSIC ICE POPS

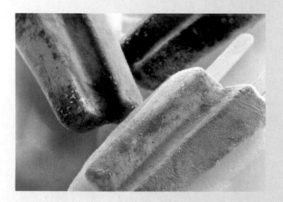

Browse the frozen-foods section of your local supermarket for an ice pop that tastes good but doesn't have added sugar or artificial dyes, and you could very well get brain freeze. Even brands touting whole-fruit blends will typically have at least one sneaky source of added sugar.

Not mine. I created a chilly treat using pure fruit (fresh or frozen—your choice) to sweeten your day. I even top off my ice pops with a hidden vegetable. Trust me, your finicky friends (and kids) will rave, and they'll have no idea they're eating something healthy.

Joy Food

45 CALORIES

BERRY ICE POPS

makes 7 servings

While I'm all about helping kids learn to love their veggies, sometimes hiding them in a treat is the way to go. These refreshing pops get their sweetness (and they *are* sweet) naturally from bananas and berries. And while I snuck in some spinach for extra nutrition, believe it or not, you won't even taste it. I'm confident because I've tested these out on the pickiest of kids (and spouses), and they didn't suspect a thing. The overwhelming response? Another ice pop, please!

> 1 ripe banana
> 1½ cups fresh or frozen blueberries
> ½ cup sliced fresh or frozen strawberries
> ½ cup low-fat milk
> 1 cup baby spinach leaves, loosely packed

Combine all the ingredients in a blender and puree until completely mixed. Add a bit more milk if the mixture is too thick.

Pour about ⅓ cup of the mixture into each of 7 ice pop molds, and freeze for at least 5 hours or overnight.

---

nutrition information PER SERVING
45 calories ▪ 1 g protein ▪ 0 g total fat (0 g unsaturated, 0 g saturated) ▪ 0 mg cholesterol ▪ 10 g carbs ▪ 2 g fiber
6 g total sugar (6 g natural, 0 g added) ▪ 10 mg sodium

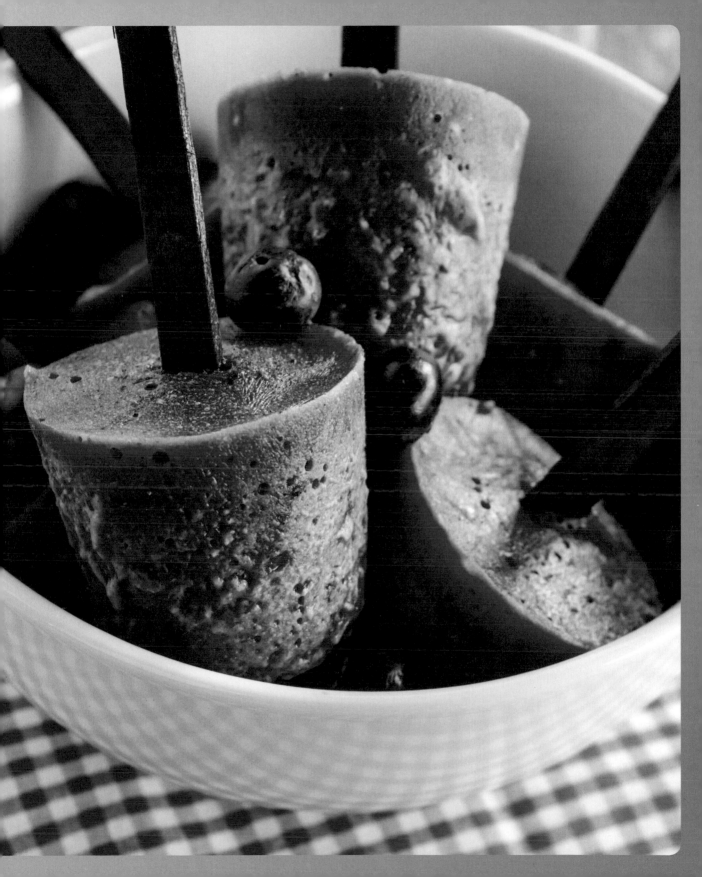

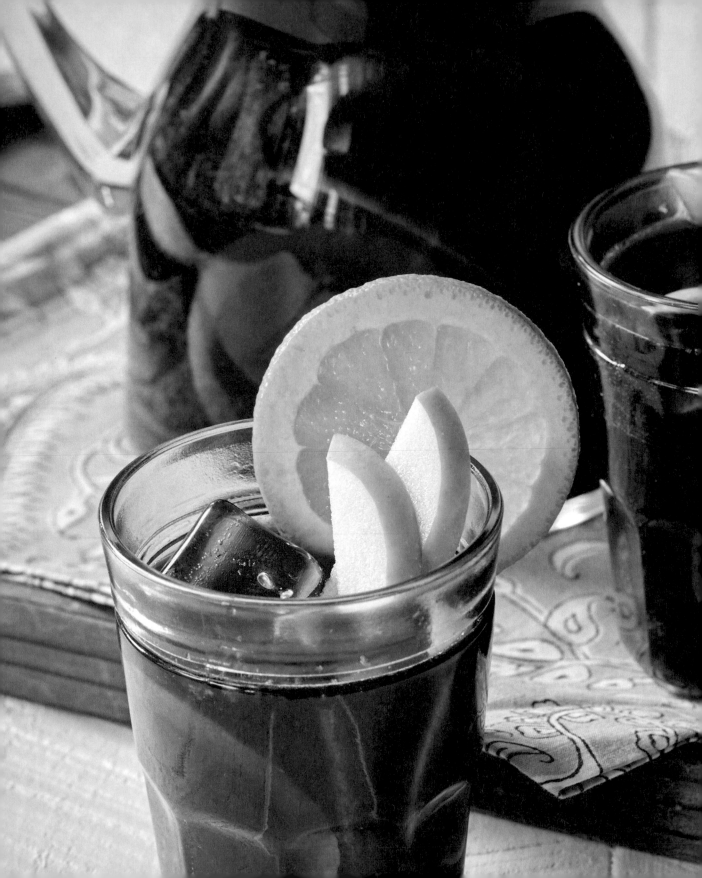

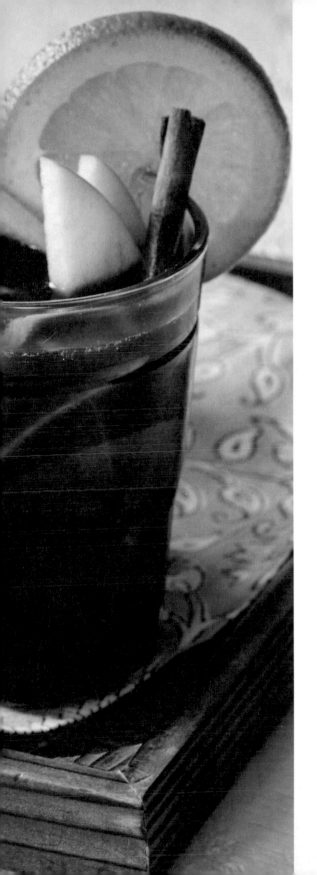

Chapter 8

CREATIVE COCKTAILS, MOCKTAILS, AND BEVERAGES

It's all too easy to slurp down hundreds of empty calories without even realizing it. Soda and other sugary sips, coffee and all its add-ons, signature cocktails, and more—these beverages do little to satisfy your appetite but have a huge impact on your health and waistline.

Fortunately, I have 12 fabulous reasons to raise your glass—a dozen delicious drinks that you can whip up to celebrate a special occasion, warm up on a cold day, or simply quench your thirst. No reason to waste your calories or cash when you can mix your own refreshing versions of these classic drinks at home. Cheers!

Junk Food

PUMPKIN SPICE LATTE

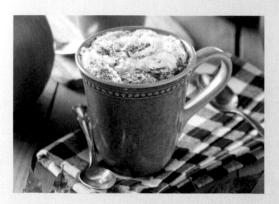

Nothing says fall like a big chunky sweater, except maybe a warm, cozy, pumpkin spice latte from the local coffee shop. But if you enjoy a bunch of these delicious seasonal sips each week, your favorite oversized sweater will soon become undersized and uncomfortable. Eek.

No need to skip sipping, though. Instead, try my DIY simple and slim substitute.

Joy Food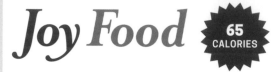

PUMPKIN SPICE LATTE

makes 1 serving

Get ready for fall by making your own pumpkin-y treat at home. This soothing beverage will really hit the spot. Plus, you'll save sugar, calories, and some cash, too. *Boom.*

> ¼ teaspoon vanilla extract
> ½ cup skim milk
> 1 cup brewed hot coffee
> 1 teaspoon sugar
> ¼ teaspoon pumpkin pie spice

Combine the vanilla and milk in a small bowl and microwave until very hot, about 50 seconds.

Pour the vanilla-milk mixture into a mug (see note) with the brewed hot coffee and stir in the sugar and pumpkin pie spice.

Note: If you enjoy a foam finish, save about 3 tablespoons of the hot vanilla-milk mixture and whisk for about 1 minute until foamy. Pour on top of your latte.

---

nutrition information PER SERVING
65 calories • 4.5 g protein • 0 g total fat (0 g unsaturated, 0 g saturated) • 0 mg cholesterol • 11 g carbs • 0 g fiber 10 g total sugar (6 g natural, 4 g added) • 65 mg sodium

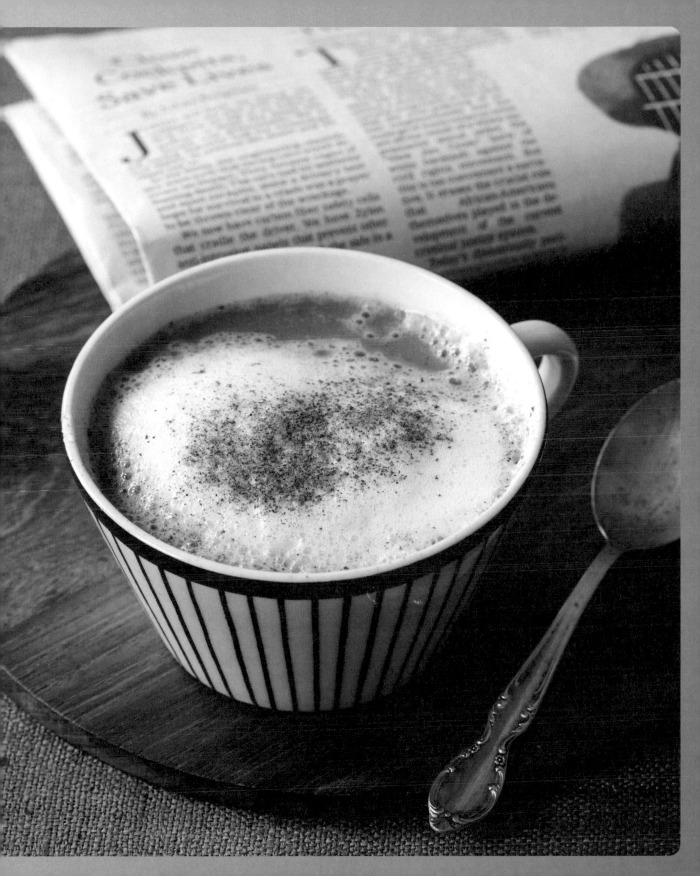

Junk Food

160 CALORIES

PEACH ICED TEA

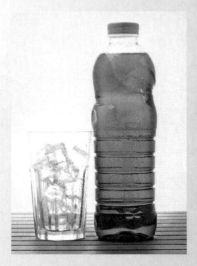

Sweetened tea drinks—just like soda—are saturated with sugar, which can tamper with mood and energy levels, elevate cholesterol and blood sugar, aggravate inflammation, and cause weight gain. What's more, liquid calories are nowhere near as satisfying as food. Study after study shows just how harmful sugar-sweetened beverages can be for our waistline and our health. Don't sip down all that unnecessary stuff!

Here's a flavorful alternative: quench your thirst with my zero-cal iced tea instead.

> **CHOOSE IT TO LOSE IT** Replace your daily sweetened iced tea (peach or other flavor) with this Peach Iced Tea and you'll save more than 58,000 calories annually, which could help you shed more than 16 pounds in a year.

Joy Food

0 CALORIES

PEACH-RASPBERRY ICED TEA

makes 8 servings

This refreshing twist on fruity tea is the perfect solution if you're looking to jazz up plain old water. It's also a great option to help cool you down on a stifling hot day. Plus, it has no calories, carbs, sugar, or fat—this is one time you'll love being a total zero.

   4 peach tea bags
   4 raspberry tea bags

Add the tea bags to a 2-quart (8-cup) pitcher and fill it about one-third of the way with boiling water.

Steep for 5 minutes, then remove the tea bags. Fill the rest of the pitcher with cold water. Serve over lots and lots of ice.

nutrition information PER SERVING

0 calories ▪ 0 g protein ▪ 0 g total fat (0 g unsaturated, 0 g saturated) ▪ 0 mg cholesterol ▪ 0 g carbs ▪ 0 g fiber 0 g total sugar (0 g natural, 0 g added) ▪ 0 mg sodium

> **TASTY TWIST** I love trying this with all sorts of tea flavors, so feel free to experiment. You'll be surprised what you can create. Also, elevate the presentation by floating fresh or frozen sliced peaches and raspberries in your pitcher or glass.

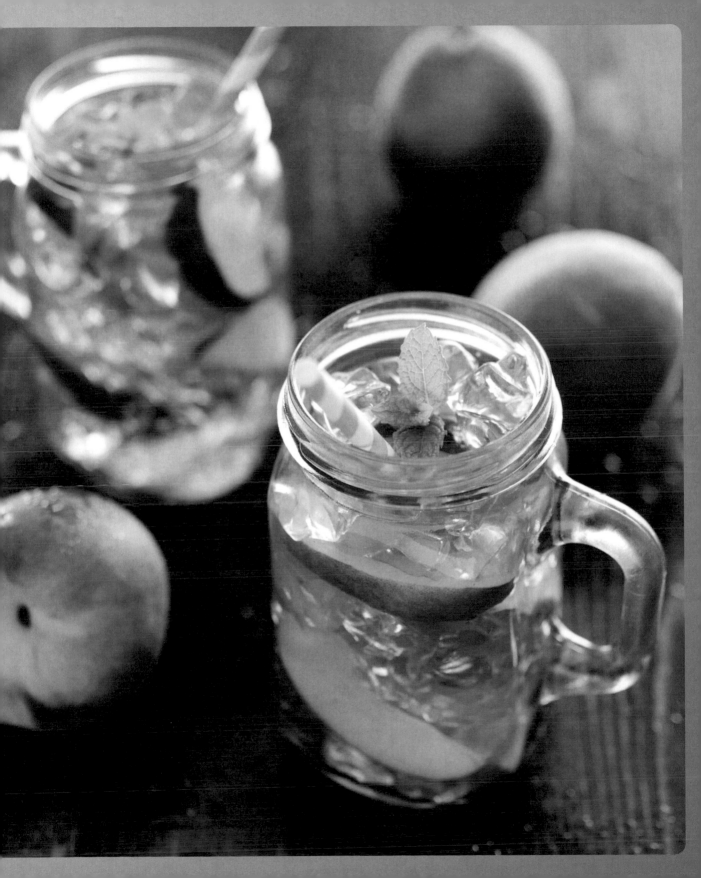

Junk Food

450 CALORIES

HOT CHOCOLATE

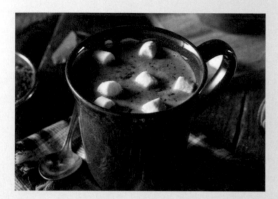

I don't know about you, but when the cold winter months settle in, I love to warm up with a steamy mug of hot cocoa. However, if you're not careful, that cup of whole milk mixed with rich chocolate and whatever toppings you drop in your cup (marshmallows, whipped cream, and so on) could really cost you—as much as 450 calories per mug at some coffee shops. You'd be better off slapping on a pair of fuzzy mittens—it's not nearly as tasty, but hey, at least it's a trimmer way to get toasty.

Or you could try a cup of my dark chocolate hot cocoa. It's good to the last drop!

Joy Food

185 CALORIES

DARK HOT CHOCOLATE

makes 3 servings

Curl up on the couch with this slim-style hot cocoa. The skim milk adds a blast of bone-strengthening calcium, and the dark chocolate enriches your mug with heart-healthy antioxidants. Of course, I couldn't leave out the sugar, but I substantially reduced the amount compared to what you'll find in your coffee-shop version. I think you'll agree it's the perfect amount for sweet satisfaction.

> 3 cups skim milk
> 2 tablespoons sugar
> 1 teaspoon vanilla extract
> Pinch of kosher salt or coarse sea salt
> 3 tablespoons dark chocolate chips

Heat the milk in a small saucepan over medium-high heat until it is hot and starting to steam, about 5 minutes. Remove the saucepan from the heat.

Add the sugar, vanilla, salt, and chocolate chips, and whisk until the chocolate is completely melted.

Pour 1 cup of hot cocoa into each of 3 mugs.

---

nutrition information PER 1-CUP SERVING
185 calories ▪ 9 g protein ▪ 5 g total fat (2 g unsaturated, 3 g saturated) ▪ 5 mg cholesterol ▪ 30 g carbs ▪ 1 g fiber 28 g total sugar (12 g natural, 16 g added) ▪ 150 mg sodium

> **TASTY TWIST** Elevate your hot cocoa by adding 8 mini marshmallows (10 calories), a generous squirt of canned whipped topping (15 calories), and 1 teaspoon of dark chocolate shavings (15 calories).

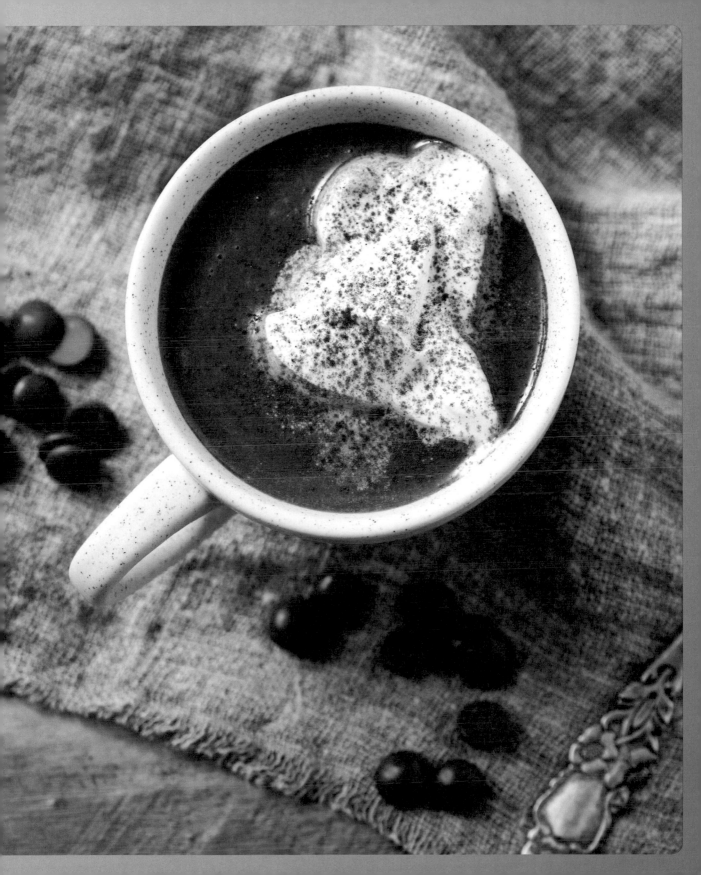

Junk Food

160 CALORIES

CHERRY SODA

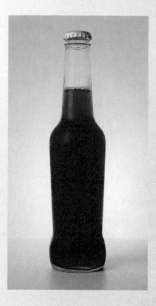

Addicted to soda? You're not alone! Many people crave the sweetness, the fizz, and the flavor. But as you probably already know, these beverages are loaded with added sugar and extra calories, and provide little to no nutrition. Just look at cherry cola—a 12-ounce can of the sweet stuff contains, on average, 160 calories and 43 grams of sugar. That's nearly 11 teaspoons of straight sugar—more than the daily amount recommended by health organizations.

Instead, whip up my refreshing and subtly sweet Cherry Soda and slightly downsize your portion. You'll get the same fizzy flavor for less than half the calories . . . without a drop of added sugar.

Joy Food

75 CALORIES

CHERRY SODA

makes 5 servings

Create your own cherry soda right at home—and save yourself a ton of sugar—by pairing carbonation from seltzer with frozen sweet cherries and tart cherry juice. It will not only satisfy your soda cravings but also ease your aches and pains: tart cherry juice and ginger have been shown to have strong anti-inflammatory properties.

> 2 cups no-sugar-added tart cherry juice blend
> 1 cup frozen pitted sweet cherries
> ½ cup lemon juice
> ¼ teaspoon ground ginger, or up to
>   1 tablespoon grated fresh ginger
> 3 cups cherry-flavored sparkling water
>   or seltzer

Puree the cherry juice, frozen cherries, lemon juice, and ginger in a blender until completely smooth.

Transfer to a large pitcher and add the sparkling water and plenty of ice.

---

nutrition information PER 8-OUNCE SERVING
75 calories ▪ 1 g protein ▪ 0 g total fat (0 g unsaturated, 0 g saturated) ▪ 0 mg cholesterol ▪ 19 g carbs ▪ 1 g fiber 15 g total sugar (15 g natural, 0 g added) ▪ 0 mg sodium

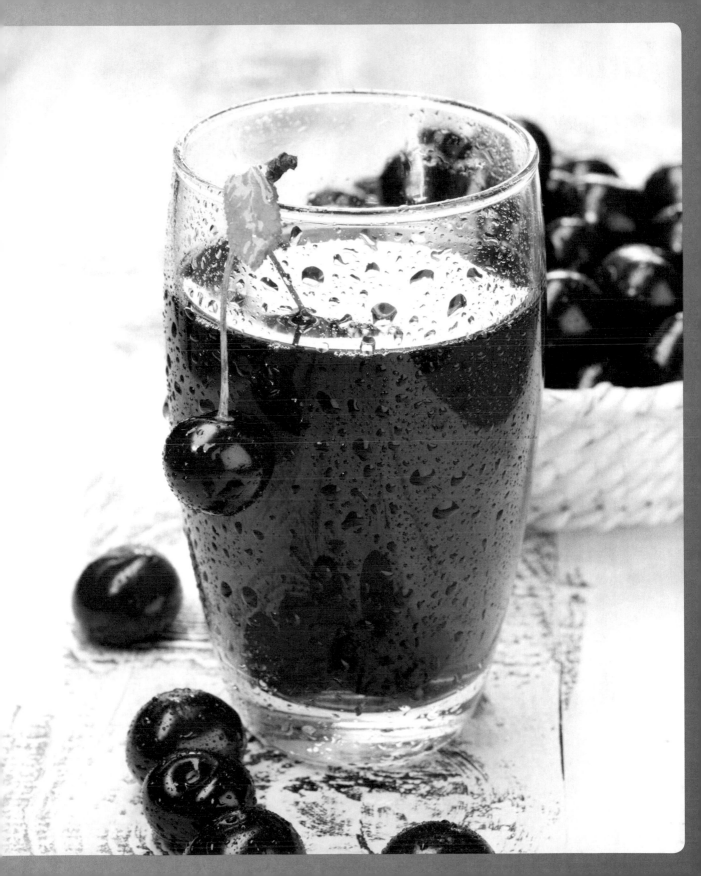

Junk Food

180 CALORIES

WATERMELON SLUSH

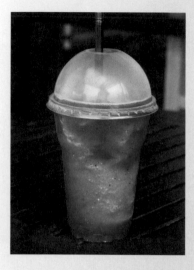

A watermelon slush may feel light and go down smoothly, but beware: a small portion can have about 180 calories and more than 12 teaspoons of straight sugar. Order a medium, and you could be ingesting 71 grams (about 18 teaspoons) of sugar . . . from just one drink!

My refreshing watermelon spritzer offers the same yummy flavors in a healthier form. Skip the drive-through and start blending.

Joy Food

36 CALORIES

WATERMELON SPRITZER

makes 8 servings

Talk about the perfect summer beverage. Watermelon, the star ingredient, is 92 percent water, making it the ultimate hydrating fruit. Add in a hint of ginger, as well as refreshing mint and some sparkly seltzer, and you've got yourself a pretty special beverage. In the mood for a cocktail? Simply add a shot of rum to each glass and enjoy an adult evening with friends.

> 6 cups watermelon cubes
> Juice of 1 lime
> 2 tablespoons grated fresh ginger, or
>   1½ teaspoons ground ginger
> 2 sprigs mint, plus more for garnish (optional)
> Ice
> 8 cups seltzer
> 8 wedges watermelon (optional)

Add the watermelon, lime juice, ginger, and 2 sprigs of mint to a blender. Blend until thoroughly mixed.

Pour the mixture into a pitcher with ice cubes and add the seltzer. Pour 1 cup into each glass and garnish each with a wedge of watermelon and an additional sprig of mint, if desired.

nutrition information PER 1-CUP SERVING
36 calories ▪ 1 g protein ▪ 0 g total fat (0 g unsaturated, 0 g saturated) ▪ 0 mg cholesterol ▪ 9 g carbs ▪ 0.5 g fiber 7 g total sugar (7 g natural, 0 g added) ▪ 0 mg sodium

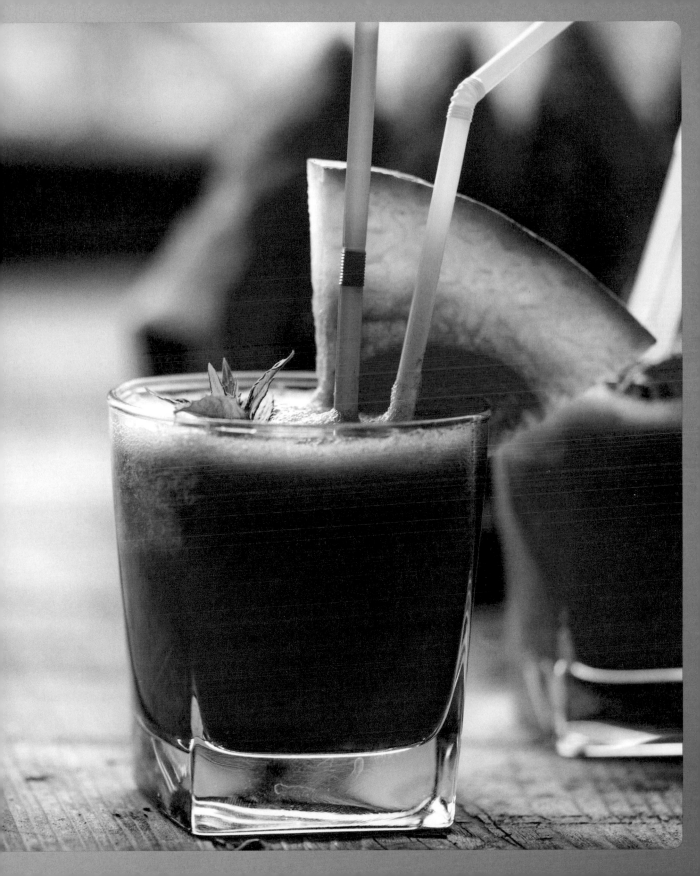

Junk Food

290 CALORIES

FROZEN MOCHA COFFEE

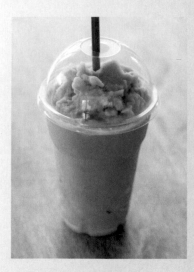

Like your coffee frozen and frothy? A typical small mocha beverage at popular coffee shops can have as many as 290 calories and 42 grams of sugar. How's that for a jolt?!

If you're looking for a lighter way to get the same flavor fix, try my Iced Mocha Coffee—it's a trim trifecta of chocolate, coffee, and caffeine. You can even double up on the portion size and still clock in with fewer than 150 calories.

Joy Food

72 CALORIES

ICED MOCHA COFFEE

makes 1 serving

This simple and delicious concoction will give you a dose of caffeine while your taste buds do a happy dance. It's a perfect midafternoon pick-me-up.

- ½ cup brewed cold coffee
- ¼ cup skim milk
- 1 tablespoon chocolate syrup
- 4 to 5 ice cubes

Place all ingredients in a blender and process until smooth and frothy.

nutrition information PER SERVING
72 calories ▪ 2.5 g protein ▪ 0 g total fat (0 g unsaturated, 0 g saturated) ▪ 0 mg cholesterol ▪ 15 g carbs ▪ 0 g fiber 12.5 g total sugar (3 g natural, 9.5 g added) ▪ 36 mg sodium

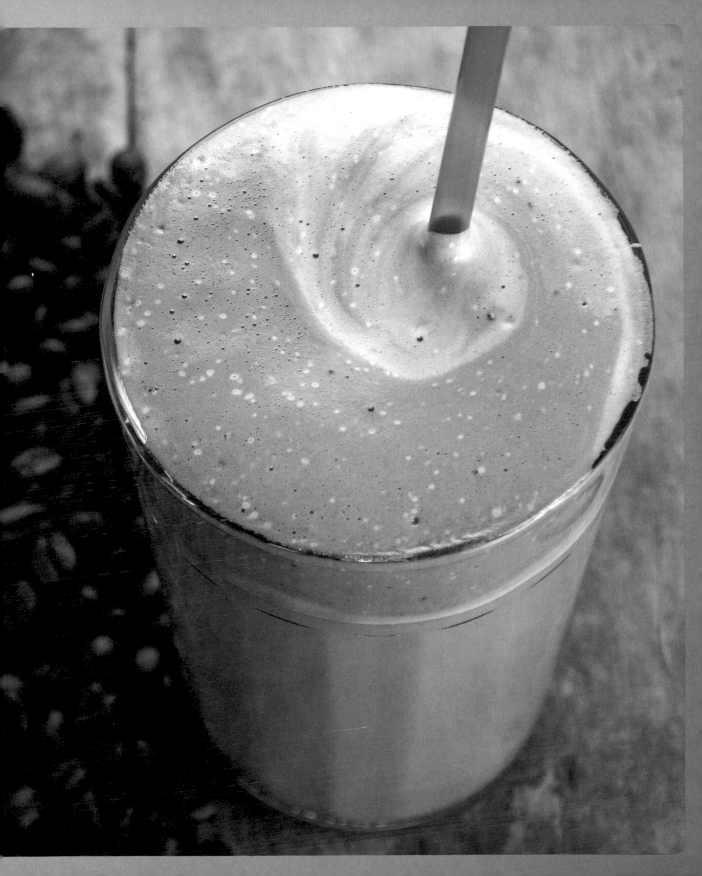

Junk Food

EGGNOG

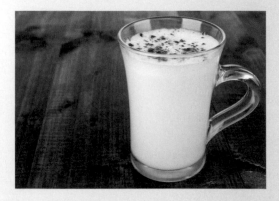

Traditional eggnog, made with cream, whole milk, egg yolks, and sugar, typically contains more than 350 calories and 12 grams of saturated fat per cup. Bah humbug!

My slim-style version satisfies your craving but with less than half the calories—and a fraction of the fat. Cheers to health-ifying a holiday beverage classic.

Joy Food

EGGNOG

makes 5 servings

Hosting a holiday party? Whip up a batch of this deliciously light eggnog for your guests. They'll love the taste and the fact that it won't break the calorie bank.

> 5 cups skim milk
> One 3.4-ounce package instant vanilla pudding
> ¾ teaspoon rum extract
> ½ teaspoon fresh nutmeg
> Cinnamon (optional)
> 5 cinnamon sticks (optional)

Put all the ingredients in a blender and process until mixed.

Pour the eggnog into a pitcher and refrigerate for about 20 minutes to allow it to set. (The longer you leave it to chill, the thicker it gets. If it's too thick before serving, simply put it back in the blender and add milk, a little bit at a time, while blending to make sure you get the consistency you want.)

Garnish each glass with a sprinkle of extra nutmeg and cinnamon, plus a cinnamon stick, if desired.

---

nutrition information PER 8-OUNCE SERVING
157 calories ▪ 8 g protein ▪ 0 g total fat (0 g unsaturated, 0 g saturated) ▪ 5 mg cholesterol ▪ 30 g carbs ▪ 0 g fiber 30 g total sugar (12 g natural, 18 g added) ▪ 380 mg sodium

> **TASTY TWIST** If you really want to get into the holiday spirit, add 1 ounce of real rum to each glass for an extra 65 calories.

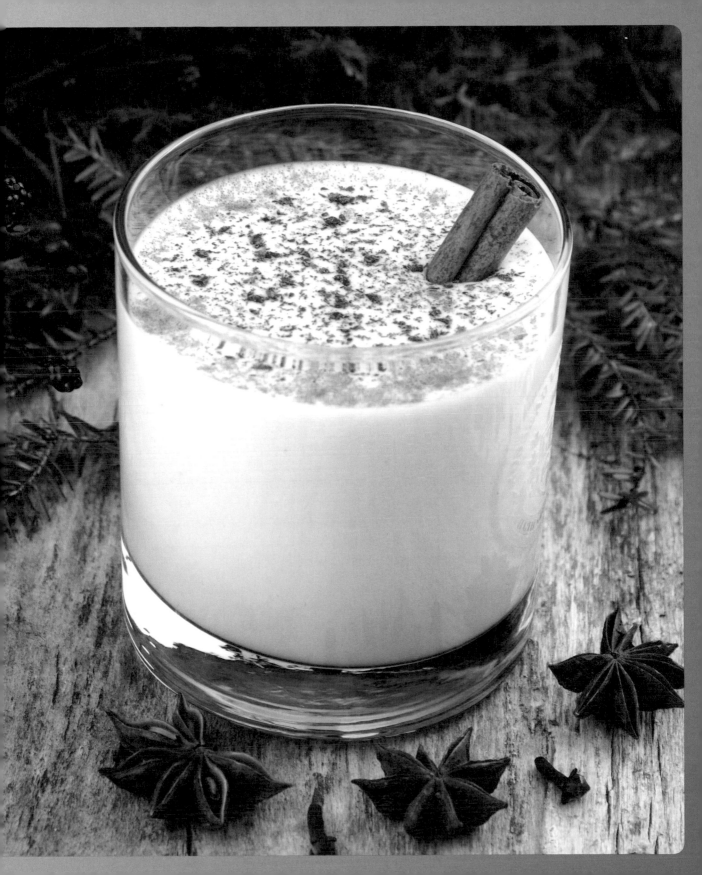

Junk Food

LONG ISLAND ICED TEA

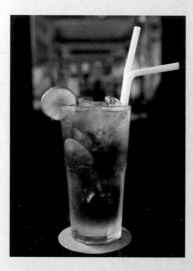

Looking for a refreshing cocktail? Beware: Some drinks may cool you off, but they can also weigh you down. Take your typical Long Island iced tea, which contains five different types of alcohol—vodka, gin, rum, tequila, and triple sec—as well as sweet-and-sour mix and cola. It can pack as many as 440 calories per glass.

I created a slimmer sip while on vacation with my extended family (all 29 of us!) in Stockbridge, Massachusetts. It has become our cocktail of choice when we're relaxing in the Berkshires. I'm hoping you love it as much as we do. Bottoms up.

Joy Food

BERKSHIRE ICED TEA

makes 1 serving

Not only did I give this classic drink a new name (after one of my favorite places on Earth), but I also gave it a healthy spin, thanks to the grapefruit juice (*ciao*, cola!) and lemon-ginger tea bag (so long, sweet-and-sour mix). Of course, you can easily prepare a virgin version instead (skip the alcohol and it's just 25 calories). Whichever you choose, kick back and sip on.

> 1 lemon-ginger tea bag
> ¼ cup 100% grapefruit juice
> 1 tablespoon vodka
> 1 tablespoon rum
> 1 wedge fresh grapefruit (optional)
> 1 sprig mint (optional)

Place the tea bag in 1 cup of boiling water and steep for 5 minutes. Remove tea bag and allow tea to cool in fridge.

Once cool, mix in the grapefruit juice, vodka, and rum.

Stir and add ice.

Garnish with grapefruit wedge and mint, if desired.

---

nutrition information PER SERVING
90 calories ▪ 0 g protein ▪ 0 g total fat (0 g unsaturated, 0 g saturated) ▪ 0 mg cholesterol ▪ 6 g carbs ▪ 0 g fiber 6 g total sugar (6 g natural, 0 g added) ▪ 0 mg sodium

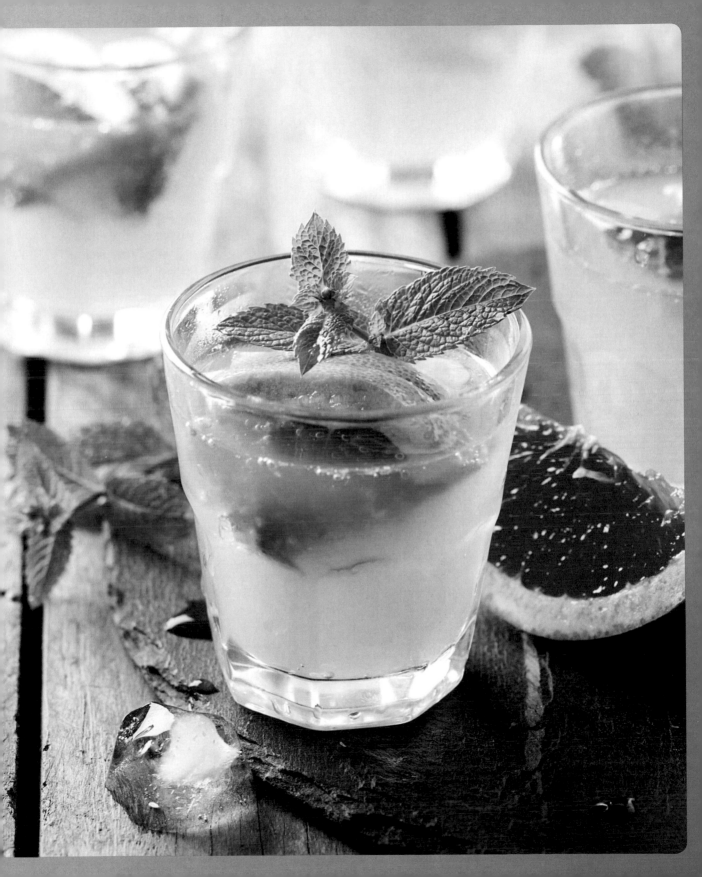

Junk Food

PIÑA COLADA

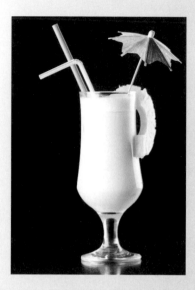

Piña coladas go hand in hand with vacation. The indulgent frozen tropical treat is the ultimate beach beverage. But with about 500 calories per glass, don't think you can sip away and keep that bikini body.

My slimmed-down version features only four ingredients and skips the sugary mixes, fruit juice, and syrupy fruit. As a result, it clocks in at a fraction of the calories. Beach and pool party perfection!

Joy Food

PIÑA COLADA

makes 2 servings

Yes, I like piña coladas. (You're totally finishing that thought with something about the rain . . . aren't you?) I'm happy to share a simple way to get the same delicious tropical flavor without the sky-high calorie count. Enjoy it spiked for 175 calories, or blend up a virgin version for just 130 calories.

> 1½ cups frozen pineapple chunks
> ¾ cup canned light coconut milk (see note)
> 3 to 5 ice cubes
> 1½ ounces rum
> 1 to 2 drops coconut extract (optional)
> 2 wedges fresh pineapple (optional)

Add all the ingredients to a blender and process until smooth and creamy.

Pour the piña coladas into glasses and garnish each with a pineapple wedge, if desired.

Note: Because canned coconut milk tends to separate, make sure to shake the can well before you open it.

---

nutrition information PER SERVING
175 calories ▪ 1 g protein ▪ 6 g total fat (1.5 g unsaturated, 4.5 g saturated) ▪ 0 mg cholesterol ▪ 17.5 g carbs ▪ 2 g fiber 13 g total sugar (13 g natural, 0 g added) ▪ 25 mg sodium

> **TASTY TWIST** To make these even more coconutty and delicious, add 2 tablespoons of shredded, unsweetened coconut before blending. It adds only 35 calories but it will taste even more tropical.

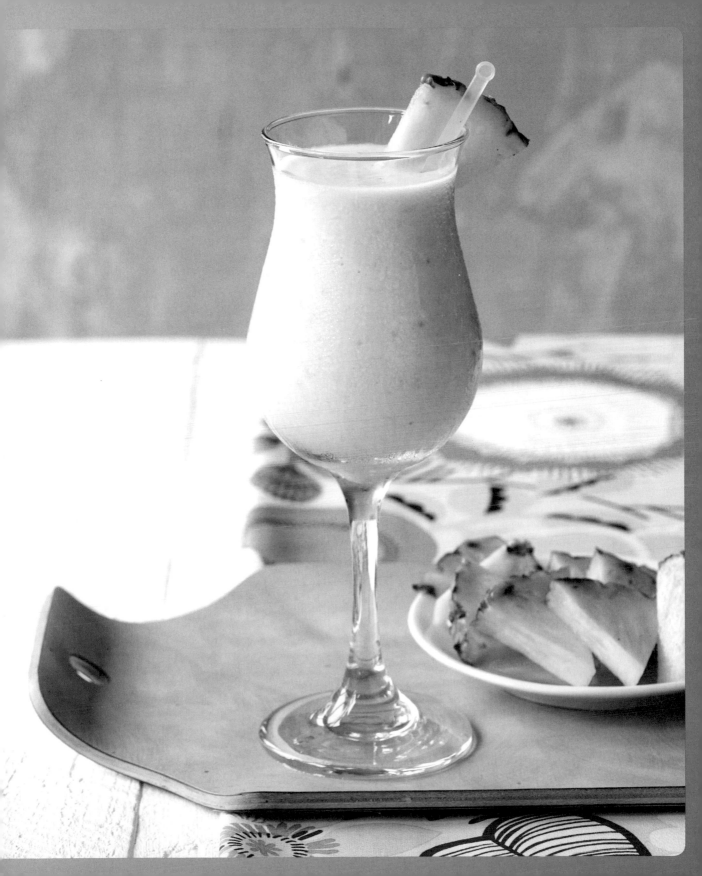

Junk Food **220 CALORIES**

SANGRIA

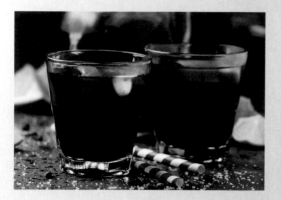

Let's face it—there aren't many ways to improve on a glass of wine. I think we can all agree on the fact that it's pretty fabulous as it is. Unless you're talking about sangria, which involves infusing wine with fresh fruit, a sweetener of some sort, and usually a bit of brandy. But all these delicious extras can add calories and sugar—a glass will typically cost you 220 calories, and in some instances more, depending on the amount of sweetener added (for example, fruit juice, punch, soda, and simple syrup).

I've slimmed down sangria by adding flavored seltzer (0 calories) and cutting back on fruit juice and other sweetened liquids. Grab some friends and start sipping.

Joy Food **170 CALORIES**

SPARKLING SANGRIA
makes 6 servings

Whip up a batch of this fruity sangria for your next get-together and be ready to share the recipe with your guests. The red wine donates heart-healthy antioxidants, and you'll get a produce perk from the sliced apples and oranges. Truly, it's a party in a pitcher.

> 1 bottle (750 ml) red table wine
> ¾ cup 100% orange juice
> ¼ cup orange-flavored liqueur (such as Cointreau or Grand Marnier)
> 2 oranges, sliced
> 1 Granny Smith apple, sliced
> 1 cinnamon stick
> ½ liter chilled seltzer (pomegranate, cranberry, berry, or orange flavored)

Combine the red wine, orange juice, orange liqueur, fruit, and cinnamon stick in a large pitcher. Chill this mixture in the refrigerator for at least 4 hours, preferably overnight.

Remove the cinnamon stick and add the seltzer into the pitcher right before serving. Stir all of the contents and pour into glasses.

---

nutrition information PER 8-OUNCE SERVING
170 calories • 1 g protein • 0 g total fat (0 g unsaturated, 0 g saturated) • 0 mg cholesterol • 15 g carbs • 1.5 g fiber 7.5 g total sugar (7.5 g natural, 0 g added) • 5 mg sodium

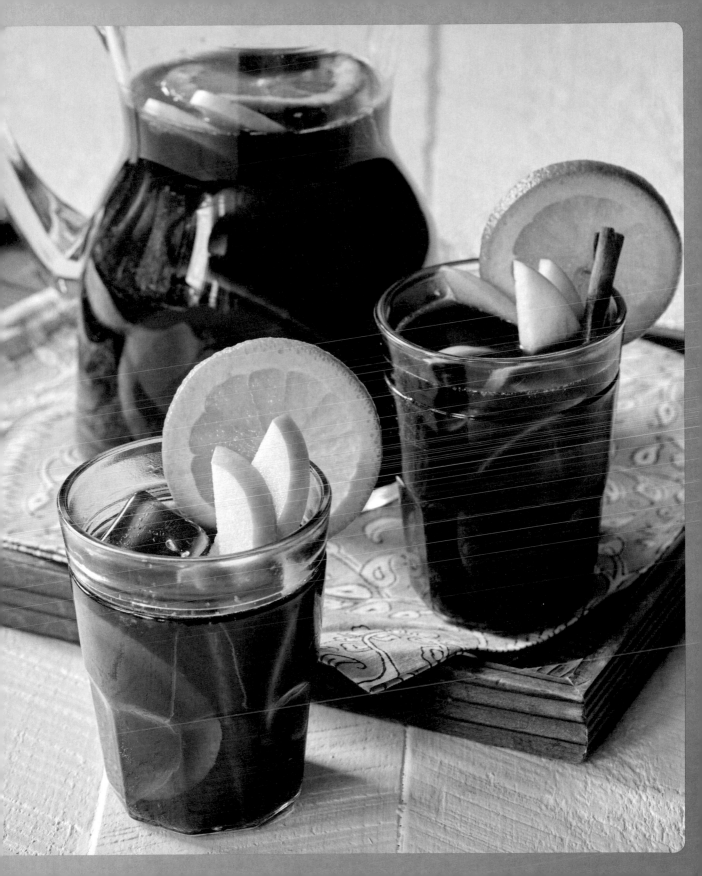

Junk Food

215 CALORIES

MOJITO

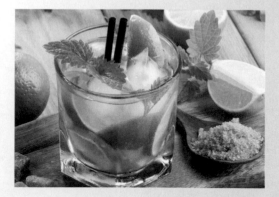

The mixture of mint and citrus is a mouthwatering marriage, but stir the sugar and rum into the signature cocktail and you wind up with a bunch of extra calories. On average, you'll be sipping 215 per beverage. Not bad, but we can do better.

My Blueberry Mojito contains fresh fruit so you get natural sweetness (with less added sugar and fewer calories) while enjoying a refreshing and delicious flavor.

Joy Food

160 CALORIES

BLUEBERRY MOJITO

makes 1 serving

This fruity mojito is the perfect summer cocktail (although you can enjoy it year-round using frozen blueberries). I take advantage of the berries' natural sweetness by muddling them with mint and lime juice to create a lower-cal drink with minimal added sugar. I personally love it with the added dash of sugar, but you can certainly omit it for a lower-calorie bevvy that clocks in at just 145 per glass.

½ cup fresh or frozen blueberries
10 fresh mint leaves
1 ounce lime juice
1 teaspoon sugar
1½ ounces light rum
½ cup ice cubes, crushed
Seltzer

If you're using frozen blueberries, let them thaw.

Muddle the blueberries, mint, lime juice, and sugar in the bottom of a glass. Add the rum and crushed ice and stir. Top with a generous splash of club soda.

---

nutrition information PER SERVING
160 calories ▪ 0.5 g protein ▪ 0 g total fat (0 g unsaturated, 0 g saturated) ▪ 0 mg cholesterol ▪ 17 g carbs ▪ 2 g fiber 11.5 g total sugar (7.5 g natural, 4 g added) ▪ 0 mg sodium

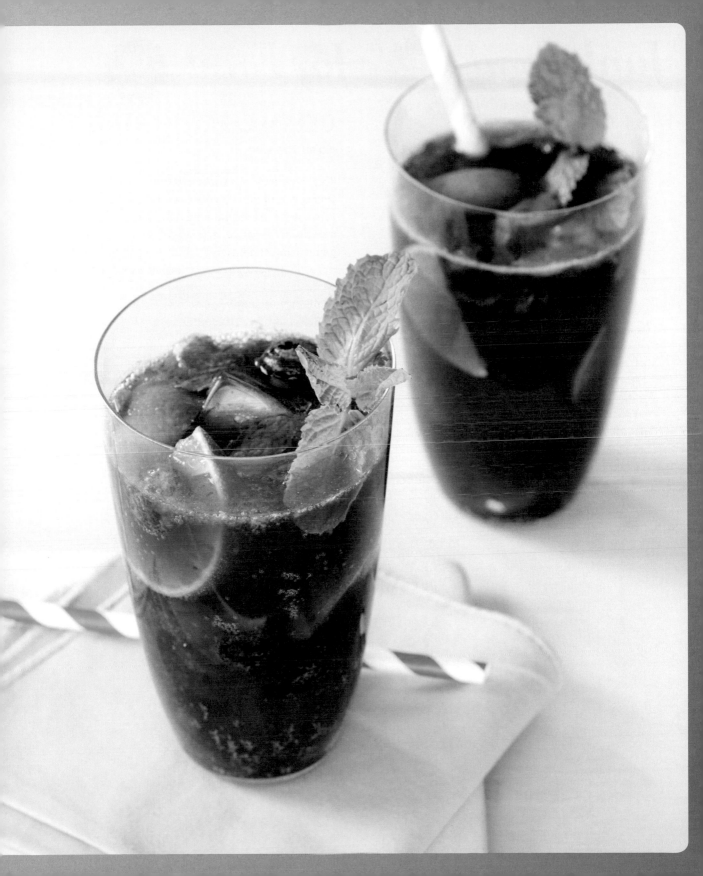

Junk Food

200 CALORIES

COSMOPOLITAN

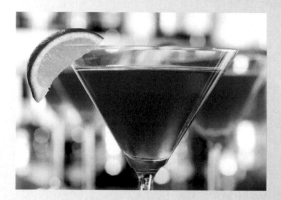

Carrie Bradshaw and the *Sex and the City* crew made the cosmopolitan popular by ordering it night after night while gallivanting around Manhattan, but there's no way you could drink it that often and still fit into your designer jeans. So curb your cosmo cravings, and instead, fill your glass with my special "Cosmopoli-trim." You can *sip and snip* without skipping a beat.

Joy Food

105 CALORIES

COSMOPOLI-TRIM

makes 1 serving

My Cosmopoli-trim has about half the alcohol of your typical fruity cocktail, so you'll be able to enjoy yourself without getting too tipsy. Sweet and tangy cranberry juice mixes with hints of lime to create a delicious signature summer drink that's refreshingly lower in sugar and calories.

> 3 ounces cranberry juice
> 2 ounces berry-flavored seltzer,
>   preferably cranberry
> 1 ounce vodka
> 1 tablespoon lime juice
> 1 lime wedge (optional)

Combine the cranberry juice, seltzer, vodka, and lime juice in a glass over ice and stir. Garnish the glass with the lime wedge, if desired.

---

nutrition information PER SERVING
105 calories ▪ 0 g protein ▪ 0 g total fat (0 g unsaturated, 0 g saturated) ▪ 0 mg cholesterol ▪ 11 g carbs ▪ 0 g fiber 10.5 g total sugar (10.5 g natural, 0 g added) ▪ 0 mg sodium

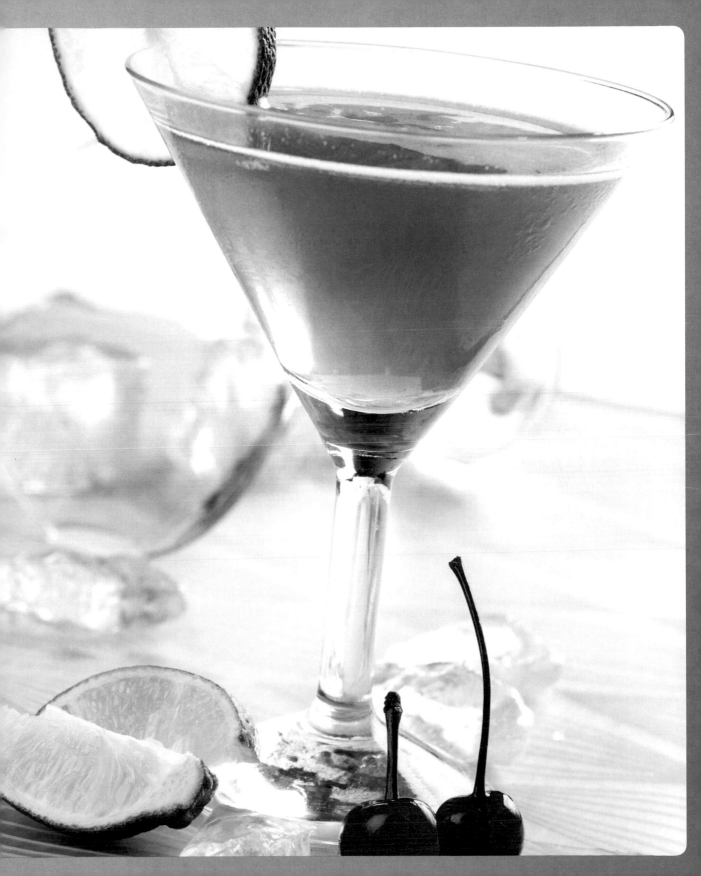

CONVERSION CHARTS

The recipes in this book use the standard United States method for measuring liquid and dry or solid ingredients (teaspoons, tablespoons, and cups). The following charts are provided to help cooks outside the U.S. successfully use these recipes. All equivalents are approximate.

Standard Cup	Fine Powder (e.g., flour)	Grain (e.g., rice)	Granular (e.g., sugar)	Liquid Solids (e.g., butter)	Liquid (e.g., milk)
1	140 g	150 g	190 g	200 g	240 ml
¾	105 g	113 g	143 g	150 g	180 ml
⅔	93 g	100 g	125 g	133 g	160 ml
½	70 g	75 g	95 g	100 g	120 ml
⅓	47 g	50 g	63 g	67 g	80 ml
¼	35 g	38 g	48 g	50 g	60 ml
⅛	18 g	19 g	24 g	25 g	30 ml

Useful Equivalents for Liquid Ingredients by Volume				
¼ tsp			1 ml	
½ tsp			2 ml	
1 tsp			5 ml	
3 tsp	1 tbsp		½ fl oz	15 ml	
	2 tbsp	⅛ cup	1 fl oz	30 ml	
	4 tbsp	¼ cup	2 fl oz	60 ml	
	5⅓ tbsp	⅓ cup	3 fl oz	80 ml	
	8 tbsp	½ cup	4 fl oz	120 ml	
	10⅔ tbsp	⅔ cup	5 fl oz	160 ml	
	12 tbsp	¾ cup	6 fl oz	180 ml	
	16 tbsp	1 cup	8 fl oz	240 ml	
	1 pt	2 cups	16 fl oz	480 ml	
	1 qt	4 cups	32 fl oz	960 ml	
			33 fl oz	1000 ml	1 l

Useful Equivalents for Dry Ingredients by Weight

(To convert ounces to grams, multiply the number of ounces by 30.)

1 oz	⅟₁₆ lb	30 g
4 oz	¼ lb	120 g
8 oz	½ lb	240 g
12 oz	¾ lb	360 g
16 oz	1 lb	480 g

Useful Equivalents for Cooking/Oven Temperatures

Process	Fahrenheit	Celsius	Gas Mark
Freeze Water	32° F	0° C	
Room Temperature	68° F	20° C	
Boil Water	212° F	100° C	
Bake	325° F	160° C	3
	350° F	180° C	4
	375° F	190° C	5
	400° F	200° C	6
	425° F	220° C	7
	450° F	230° C	8
Broil			Grill

Useful Equivalents for Length

(To convert inches to centimeters, multiply the number of inches by 2.5.)

1 in			2.5 cm	
6 in	½ ft		15 cm	
12 in	1 ft		30 cm	
36 in	3 ft	1 yd	90 cm	
40 in			100 cm	1 m

INDEX

ACKNOWLEDGMENTS

I love writing this section. It's a chance for me to show my deep appreciation toward talented colleagues and super supportive family members, all of whom have contributed to this delicious project in one way or another, and who, of course, share my passion for good food.

Heartfelt thanks to my editorial director, Donna Fennessy, who has been a serious savior during this incredible endeavor—she edits, crunches numbers, tests, juggles, problem-solves, and keeps me on a tight schedule (no small feat!). Special thanks to Tina Gowin Carlucci, my senior nutrition editor, for her invaluable input and recipe know-how. To the warm and wonderful Bob Marty for believing in my mission, on paper and on screen. To Ryan Nord, my dear friend and legal eagle. To my literary agents, Jane Dystel and Miriam Goderich, for their constant support and guidance.

To my entire NBC *Today* family, especially my girlfriends, Hoda Kotb and Kathie Lee Gifford, for being the ultimate taste testers, with or without a wine chaser. And one million thanks to Tammy Filler, along with Joanne LaMarca, for supporting this series with pure enthusiasm. Special thanks to Christine Gardner and Meredith Reis, too. Working with you ladies is just awesome.

To the rest of the all-star NBC team, including Deborah Turness, Noah Oppenheim, Don Nash, Tom Mazzarelli, Jackie Levin, Debbie Kosofsky, Minah Kathuria, Christine Cataldi, Adam Miller, Elena Nachmanoff, and the countless producers and assistants who allow me the privilege of delivering nourishing information to hungry Americans. And of course, my *Today* host friends who make my job a real pleasure: Matt Lauer, Savannah Guthrie, Al Roker, Natalie Morales, Carson Daly, Tamron Hall, Willie Geist, Erica Hill, Dylan Dreyer, and Sheinelle Jones. Also, thanks to Richard Greenberg and Steve Chung for keeping me out of trouble.

To Bianca Borges and her fab food squad (especially Alli and Tina), for always making my food sparkle on air. To Ed Helbig, April Bartlett, Ray Lutz, and the entire food/props team for all you do to make my segments run so smoothly. To Jane Weaver, Vidya Rao, and the entire gang at TODAY.com for allowing me to offer up slimming fare in the midst of calorific chaos. And to everyone in hair, makeup, wardrobe, and stage crew—you continuously enable me to shine.

To the entire Hay House Publishing group, thanks for putting together such an outstanding product. In particular, Reid Tracy and Patty Gift, for green-lighting this deliciously fun project, my tremendously talented editor, Laura Gray, and publicity director, Richelle Fredson, for helping create buzz and excitement. Many thanks to the entire production crew, including our extraordinary photographer, Lucy Schaeffer, and her top-notch team: Allison Simpson, food stylist, and Molly Fitzsimons, prop stylist. If you're tempted to bite the pages in this book because they look so delicious, that's all thanks to these three talented women. Also, huge thanks to John Ottavino and Ashley Palumbo.

Special thanks to my agents: Olivia Metzger, Katie Maloney, Stephanie Paciullo, and Jordan Solomon. And to Theresa Brown, Bethany Dicks, and Jeff Lesh.

To all those who helped with this book, whether you inspired a recipe, tweaked or tested a dish, or contributed in another valuable way to increase the yum factor—my appreciation and gratitude.

These people include Anthony Accomando, Veronica Costabile, Jessica DiStasi, Tito Dudley, Ryan Hand, Melissa King, Amanda Baker Lemein, Jessica Levin, Lauren McIlwaine, Angela Rivera, Nancy Sobel, Cristina Spano, and Lela Swartz.

To my *Nourish Snacks* family, for lending me your opinions and your taste buds whenever I needed them.

And a huge hug to everyone in my large and loving family for piling into my house on a moments notice to "taste and tell" (all 32 of you—Ellen, Artie, Carol, Vic, Ian, Jesse, Cole, Ayden, Debra, Steve, Ben, Noah, Becca, Chloe, Casey, Pam, Dan, Charlie, Cooper, Elena, Glenn, Trey, Billie, Levi, Otis, Mia, Jason, Annabelle, Zachary, Nancy, Jon, and Camron).

Infinite gratitude to my personal lifelines: my mom and dad (Ellen and Artie Schloss), my other mom and dad (Carol and Victor Bauer), my husband, Ian, and our three kids, Jesse, Cole, and Ayden Jane.

Finally, thanks to my favorite furry family member, Gatsby, for her nonstop love during tight deadlines.

Visit

JOYBAUER.com

for **FREE** information on a variety of health conditions, including diabetes, heart disease, and arthritis. Plus, get many **more delicious** *Joy Food* **recipes** and tricks to lose weight, boost energy and start feeling better today.

Want to drop a few pounds FAST?

Sign up for Joy's online subscription weight loss program and you'll get:

1. Hundreds of mouthwatering, **fuss-free,** family-friendly **recipes**

2. **Daily menus** that take all the work out of **healthy eating** (**NO** calorie-counting required!)

3. Countless **exercise videos**–from beginner to advanced

4. A supportive member **community**

5. A number of **interactive tracking tools** so you can **log** your impressive progress!

JOYBAUERWEIGHTLOSS.com

Join the party and lose your extra weight now!

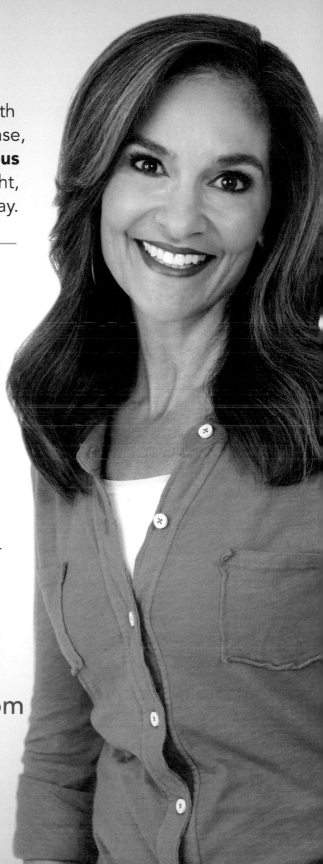

ABOUT THE AUTHOR

Joy Bauer is one of the nation's leading health authorities. As the nutrition and health expert for NBC's *TODAY* show, Joy shares reliable, practical, and straightforward advice that helps millions of Americans eat better and lead healthier, more fulfilling lives. She also hosts the program's popular "Joy Fit Club" series, which celebrates determined people who have lost more than 100 pounds through diet and exercise alone. To date, her club members have dropped an amazing 30,000 pounds collectively.

Her latest *TODAY* show series, "From *Junk Food* to *Joy Food*" was an instant hit and is the inspiration behind her new book and public television special. As a huge fan of public television, Joy was thrilled to premiere her first public television collaboration in 2014, *Joy Bauer's Food Remedies*, which continues to air across the country. And now, she's back with a brand new show, appropriately called *From Junk Food to Joy Food*, and is excited to bring many more of her tasty recipes to the public television audience.

Joy recently launched her own food line, **Nourish Snacks** (NourishSnacks.com), with a mission to provide grab-and-go treats that taste as good as they are good for you. With a wide variety of flavors—everything from dark chocolate granola clusters to chili-citrus roasted corn—all of her blends are gluten-free, dairy-free, non-GMO, and made with wholesome, nutrient-rich ingredients.

Joy is a #1 *New York Times* best-selling author with 12 books under her belt, a monthly columnist for *Woman's Day* magazine, the women's health expert for About.com, and the creator of JoyBauer.com. She is also the nutritionist for the New York City Ballet.

In the earlier part of her career, Joy was the Director of Nutrition and Fitness for the Department of Pediatric Cardiology at Mount Sinai Medical Center in New York City, as well as the clinical dietitian for their neurosurgical team. One of Joy's most rewarding experiences was creating and implementing "Heart Smart Kids," a health program for underprivileged children living in low-income communities. She also taught Anatomy and Physiology and Sports Nutrition at NYU's School of Continuing Education.

Passionate about delivering scientifically sound, realistic information, Joy received the 2010 National Media Excellence Award from the Academy of Nutrition and Dietetics and the 2012 American Society for Nutrition Science Media Award.

When Joy's not dishing out health advice or sharing delicious recipes on TV, you'll find her making a mess in her kitchen or spending quality time at home with her husband, Ian, her three kids, Jesse, Cole, and Ayden Jane, and her dog, Gatsby.

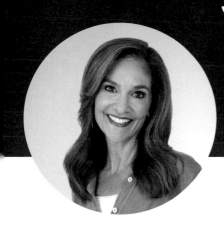

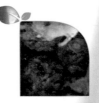

HAY HOUSE TITLES OF RELATED INTEREST

YOU CAN HEAL YOUR LIFE, the movie, starring Louise Hay & Friends
(available as a 1-DVD program and an expanded 2-DVD set)
Watch the trailer at: www.LouiseHayMovie.com

THE SHIFT, the movie, starring Dr. Wayne W. Dyer
(available as a 1-DVD program and an expanded 2-DVD set)
Watch the trailer at: www.DyerMovie.com

———————

*CULTURED FOOD FOR HEALTH: A Guide to Healing
Yourself with Probiotic Foods,* by Donna Schwenk

*THE EARTH DIET: Your Complete Guide to Living Using
Earth's Natural Ingredients,* by Liana Werner-Gray

*THE PLANT PLUS DIET SOLUTION: Personalized
Nutrition for Life,* by Joan Borysenko

*THE SPARKPEOPLE COOKBOOK: Love Your Food,
Lose the Weight,* by Meg Galvin

All of the above are available at your local bookstore,
or may be ordered by contacting Hay House (see next page).

———————

We hope you enjoyed this Hay House book. If you'd like to receive our online catalog featuring additional information on Hay House books and products, or if you'd like to find out more about the Hay Foundation, please contact:

Hay House, Inc., P.O. Box 5100, Carlsbad, CA 92018-5100
(760) 431-7695 or (800) 654-5126
(760) 431-6948 (fax) or (800) 650-5115 (fax)
www.hayhouse.com® • www.hayfoundation.org

Published and distributed in Australia by: Hay House Australia Pty. Ltd., 18/36 Ralph St., Alexandria NSW 2015 • *Phone:* 612-9669-4299 • *Fax:* 612-9669-4144 • www.hayhouse.com.au *Published and distributed in the United Kingdom by:* Hay House UK, Ltd., Astley House, 33 Notting Hill Gate, London W11 3JQ • *Phone:* 44-20-3675-2450 • *Fax:* 44-20-3675-2451 • www.hayhouse.co.uk *Published and distributed in the Republic of South Africa by:* Hay House SA (Pty), Ltd., P.O. Box 990, Witkoppen 2068 • info@hayhouse.co.za • *Published in India by:* Hay House Publishers India, Muskaan Complex, Plot No. 3, B-2, Vasant Kunj, New Delhi 110 070 • *Phone:* 91-11-4176-1620 • *Fax:* 91-11-4176-1630 • www.hayhouse.co.in • *Distributed in Canada by:* Raincoast Books, 2440 Viking Way, Richmond, B.C. V6V 1N2 • *Phone:* 1-800-663-5714 • *Fax:* 1-800-565-3770 • www.raincoast.com

---

Take Your Soul on a Vacation

Visit www.HealYourLife.com® to regroup, recharge, and reconnect with your own magnificence. Featuring blogs, mind-body-spirit news, and life-changing wisdom from Louise Hay and friends. Visit www.HealYourLife.com today!

Free e-newsletters from Hay House, the Ultimate Resource for Inspiration

Be the first to know about Hay House's dollar deals, free downloads, special offers, affirmation cards, giveaways, contests, and more!

 Get exclusive excerpts from our latest releases and videos from *Hay House Present Moments*.

 Enjoy uplifting personal stories, how-to articles, and healing advice, along with videos and empowering quotes, within *Heal Your Life*.

 Have an inspirational story to tell and a passion for writing? Sharpen your writing skills with insider tips from *Your Writing Life*.

Sign Up Now!

Get inspired, educate yourself, get a complimentary gift, and share the wisdom!

http://www.hayhouse.com/newsletters.php

Visit www.hayhouse.com to sign up today!

 HAY HOUSE

 HAYHOUSE RADIO *radio for your soul*

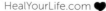 HealYourLife.com

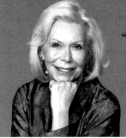
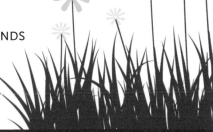